O P L

OXFORD PSYCHIATRY LIBRARY

Depression

Raymond W. Lam, MD, FRCPC

Professor and Head,
Division of Clinical Neuroscience,
Department of Psychiatry,
University of British Columbia,
Vancouver, Canada

Hiram Mok, MD, FRCPC

Clinical Associate Professor,
Department of Psychiatry,
University of British Columbia,
Vancouver, Canada

D1464350

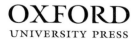

OXFORD
UNIVERSITY PRESS

OXFORD
UNIVERSITY PRESS

Great Clarendon Street, Oxford OX2 6DP

Oxford University Press is a department of the University of Oxford.
It furthers the University's objective of excellence in research, scholarship,
and education by publishing worldwide in

Oxford New York

Auckland Cape Town Dar es Salaam Hong Kong Karachi
Kuala Lumpur Madrid Melbourne Mexico City Nairobi
New Delhi Shanghai Taipei Toronto

With offices in

Argentina Austria Brazil Chile Czech Republic France Greece
Guatemala Hungary Italy Japan Poland Portugal Singapore
South Korea Switzerland Thailand Turkey Ukraine Vietnam

Oxford is a registered trade mark of Oxford University Press
in the UK and in certain other countries

Published in the United States
by Oxford University Press Inc., New York

British Library Cataloguing in Publication Data

Data available

Library of Congress Cataloging in Publication Data

Data available

Typeset by Newgen Imaging Systems (P) Ltd., Chennai, India
Printed in Italy
on acid-free paper by
LegoPrint S.p.A.

ISBN 978–0–19–921988–9

10 9 8 7 6 5 4 3 2 1

Preface

All the recent new research and knowledge about depression makes it a daunting task to summarize the vast amounts of information into manageable, yet still relevant, portions. Much of the work of this volume arose from my involvement with the Canadian Network for Mood and Anxiety Treatments (CANMAT) in developing Canadian clinical practice guidelines for depression. I am indebted to my expert CANMAT colleagues for their many hours of thought-provoking discussion about all aspects of depression and its treatment. I especially want to thank Dr Sidney H. Kennedy, Professor of Psychiatry at the University of Toronto and Chief of Psychiatry at the University Health Network, for his support and collaboration over many years.

Throughout this book we have tried to simplify the diagnosis and management of what is a complex disorder, to make the evidence relevant, and to illustrate the art and the science. Our intent is to provide a practical reference to help "at the bedside" (or, at least, at the nursing station). We hope that clinicians will find this book useful.

Raymond W. Lam, MD, FRCPC

Contents

Chapter 1

Introduction

A 36-year-old janitor who is fatigued all the time; a 24-year-old with diabetes who has stopped taking her insulin; a 40-year-old homemaker who cries and cannot cope at home; a 69-year-old seen in the emergency room with his second heart attack within 3 months; a 32-year-old executive who can't work because of headaches and insomnia; a 17-year-old high school student who cannot stop thinking about ending her life; what do all these various people have in common? They are all suffering from depression, one of the most common of all medical conditions, yet one of the most difficult to recognize.

Depression is ubiquitous, but the number and range of physical and cognitive symptoms associated with major depressive disorder (MDD) means that many people do not present with emotional symptoms. Although one in seven people will suffer psychosocial impairment from MDD, many will not be diagnosed despite repeated health care visits. And, it is not only family physicians, psychiatrists, and mental health clinicians that need to diagnose depression. The high prevalence of MDD with other medical illnesses means that other health professionals and physicians, whether internists or oncologists or surgeons or cardiologists or neurologists or any other specialist, must also recognize and manage clinical depression in their patients.

Governments and health care payers are now finally beginning to appreciate the hidden socioeconomic burden that results from MDD. Depression is a huge drain on the economy, with exceedingly high rates of disability and reduced productivity. The World Health Organization estimates that depression will be the second highest medical cause of global disability by the year 2030, second only to HIV/AIDS. The concentration and memory problems associated with depression are particularly damaging to workforces in knowledge-based industries, a major issue for many countries trying to convert from resource-based economies.

But, recognizing depression is not enough. The good news is that there are very effective treatments for depression. Evidence-based psychotherapies abound; there are many effective antidepressant medications; and several non-invasive somatic treatments also are available. With appropriate treatment, most patients are able to promptly recover from a depressive episode and return to their usual function. And, there is an explosion of new research to expand our understanding of the pathophysiology of depression, with the promise of new, more effective, and better tolerated treatments to come.

The bad news, however, is that many patients with depression are still not able to access these treatments, whether psychotherapy or new medications or new technologies. Even when available, the current systems of health care often do not achieve best practices for treating MDD, so that the "usual care" of depression is not good enough. For those patients whose depression can be regarded as a chronic or persistent condition, collaborative disease management programs that include a focus on self-management will further engage patients and clinicians to optimize care.

This book seeks to succinctly address the diagnostic and treatment issues that clinicians will encounter when dealing with patients with MDD. The principles of care for depression can be quite simple. Attention to early recognition, careful assessment, selection of appropriate treatments, and measurement-based follow-up will help our patients get the best care possible.

Key references

Adli M, Bauer M, Rush AJ. Algorithms and collaborative-care systems for depression: are they effective and why? A systematic review. *Biol Psychiatry* 2006; **59**:1029–38.

Schulberg HC, Block MR, Madonia MJ, et al. The 'usual care' of major depression in primary care practice. *Arch Fam Med* 1997; **6**(4):334–9.

Wells KB, Sherbourne C, Schoenbaum M, et al. Five-year impact of quality improvement for depression: results of a group-level randomized controlled trial. *Arch Gen Psychiatry* 2004; **61**:378–86.

Chapter 2

Epidemiology and burden

> ## Key points
>
> - Depression is a highly prevalent condition—about 1 in 7 people will experience a depressive episode during their lifetime.
> - Many people with depression will have a recurrent or chronic course, leading to substantial impairment in psychosocial function.
> - Depression is now the leading cause of disability in developed countries and the fourth leading cause worldwide.
> - The economic costs of depression are staggering, both in direct medical costs of treating depression and in indirect costs of work absence and loss of productivity.

2.1 Prevalence

2.1.1 Current trends

Depressive disorders are very common conditions as the lifetime risk for experiencing major depressive disorder (MDD) is approximately 15% (Table 2.1). Depression also contributes significantly to disability, with estimates that depression accounts for 1.3–4.4% of all disability and premature deaths worldwide. Two major epidemiological trends are occurring with respect to depressive disorders. Firstly, the lifetime risk of developing depression in those born after the Second World War is increasing, although some studies suggest this increase began as far back as 1925. Secondly, in both women and men, the age of onset for depression is becoming increasingly younger, which corresponds to the rise in psychiatric hospitalizations among adolescents.

2.1.2 Sex

The lifetime prevalence of MDD is 1.6–3.1 times more common in women than men with a greater disparity found in the USA and Western Europe. The disparity begins at the age of puberty and it is common to find worsening of depressive symptoms in women coinciding with the onset of menses. Other hypothesized causes of increased depressive episodes in women include hormonal differences, psychosocial stressors, and childbirth. The disparity between the sexes appears to be narrowing in studies involving younger cohorts and the gap also decreases after the age of 50–55 as women enter menopause.

Table 2.1 Prevalence of MDD in general populations

Location (study)	Criteria	Prevalence Rates (%)		
		Current/ 1 month	12 month	Lifetime
Europe (ESEMeD)	DSM-IV		3.9	12.8
Germany	DSM-IV	5.6	10.7	17.1
Netherlands (NEMESIS)	DSM-III-R	2.7	5.8	15.4
UK (NSPM)	ICD-10	2.1		
Canada	DSM-IV		7.4	
USA (NCS-R)	DSM-IV		6.6	16.2
USA (NCS)	DSM-III-R	4.9		17.1
Australia	DSM-IV	3.2		
Australia	ICD-10	3.3		
Japan	DSM-III-R		1.2	2.9

2.1.3 Age

In worldwide population samples aged 18–64 years, the average age for the onset of depression varies between 24 and 35 years with a mean age of 27 years. There is currently a trend of an increasingly younger age of depression onset. For example, 40% of depressed individuals have their first depressive episode prior to the age of 20, 50% have their first episode between the ages of 20 and 50, and the remaining 10% after 50 years of age.

Depressive symptoms also vary with age. Childhood depression tends to involve more somatic complaints combined with irritability and social withdrawal; adolescents experience more "atypical" features of depression (e.g., overeating, hypersomnia, etc.), while elderly depressed patients are most likely to have depressive features of melancholia (e.g., loss of interest or pleasure, lack of reactivity, etc.).

2.2 Course and prognosis

2.2.1 Course

About half of the individuals with first-episode depression experience a prodromal period during which significant depressive symptoms are present. These symptoms, which could have been present for weeks to years prior to diagnosis, include anxiety and other mild depressive symptoms. The length of an untreated depressive episode varies from 4 to 30 weeks for a mild-moderate depression, while severe episodes have an average length of 6–8 months. Nearly 25% of individuals with severe depressive episodes will endure symptoms for more than 12 months. Treated depressive episodes last on average 3 months; however, stopping antidepressants prior to 3 full months of use almost always results in the return of symptoms.

2.2.2 Prognosis

For many patients, MDD can be a chronic, relapsing illness. Relapse within the first 6 months of recovery occurs in 25% of patients, 58% will relapse within the first 5 years, and 85% will relapse within 15 years of initial recovery. Moreover, those individuals that have had two previous depressive episodes have a 70% probability of a third, and having three previous depressive episodes incurs a 90% likelihood of relapse. As the disease progresses, the interval between depressive episodes becomes shorter and the severity of each episode becomes greater. Over a 20-year span, depressive recurrences occur on average five to six times.

A significant proportion of depressed individuals remain chronically ill with varying levels of symptoms. About two-thirds of patients with a major depressive episode will fully recover, while one-third of depressed patients will either only partially recover or remain chronically ill. In a study of patients at 1 year post-MDD diagnosis, 40% had recovered with no symptoms of depression, 20% continued to have residual symptoms but did not meet the criteria for MDD, whereas 40% were still in a major depressive episode. Those individuals that continue to have residual depressive symptoms are at a high risk of relapse, suicide, poor psychosocial functioning, and higher mortality from other medical conditions. In addition to depression, 5–10% of individuals who have experienced a major depressive episode will subsequently have a manic or mixed episode indicative of bipolar disorder.

Numerous studies have focused on prognostic indicators that have a predictive value in terms of the recovery rate and relapse probability in depressed individuals (Box 2.1).

2.3 Burden of illness

2.3.1 Disability and death

Depression causes substantial impairment in daily functioning. Social functioning decreases in correlation with increasing depressive severity as 18% of patients with minor depression had major problems with daily interactions, compared to 52% of patients with seven to nine symptoms of a major depressive episode. In general, depression has been found to increase the risk of social disability 23-fold over the general population.

> **Box 2.1 Prognostic indicators of a prolonged course to recovery in patients with MDD**
>
> - Severe depressive episode
> - Long duration of depressive episode (>6 months)
> - Presence of comorbid illness
> - Presence of psychotic features
> - Early age of onset
> - Alcohol or drug abuse
> - History of prior psychiatric illness (e.g., previous depressions or anxiety disorder)
> - Three or more prior hospitalizations
> - Poor social support, poor family functioning, and low family income
> - Low level of functioning for 5 years prior to illness

Similarly, depressed patients have a two times greater overall mortality risk than the general population due to direct (e.g., suicide) and indirect (e.g., medical illness) causes. The risk of death by suicide increases 26-fold in depressed individuals. However, the lifetime prevalence of suicide for depressed individuals is 2.2% and suicide represents only 1% of reported deaths related to depression.

Depressed patients are at a 1.8 times greater risk of developing a medical illness 1 year post-diagnosis. In particular, hospitalized depressed patients with comorbid cardiovascular disease are at a significantly increased risk for myocardial infarction and death for 10 years post-hospitalization. For example, depressed patients with unstable angina are at a three times greater risk of death than non-depressed individuals. The increased risk of cardiovascular death likely is due to both direct physiological effects (e.g., reduced heart rate variability, increased platelet aggregation, etc.) and indirect effects (e.g., poor compliance with medications, drug and alcohol abuse, etc.) of depression (see Chapter 9).

2.3.2 **Socioeconomic costs**
As of 2000, depression was the leading cause of disability in developed countries, and the fourth leading cause of disability worldwide, representing 12% of all years lived with disability worldwide (Figure 2.1). The World Health Organization predicts that by 2030 depression will be the second leading cause of disability worldwide, behind only HIV/AIDS.

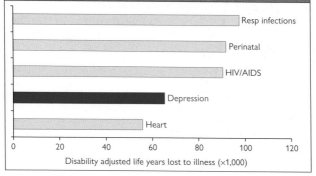

Figure 2.1 The WHO Global Burden of Disease Study. In 2000, depression ranked fourth in total disability worldwide

In terms of work productivity, those suffering with depression are three to four times more likely to take sick days off work than non-depressed individuals. In a US survey, the salary-equivalent productivity loss attributed to depressive absenteeism (average US$182–395) approached the estimated cost of treating depression. Studies have also found that employers, on the whole, have negative stigma toward mental illness and are less likely to hire depressed individuals based on expectations of substandard work performance. In fact, depressed individuals have a perceived increase in self-rated productivity when they experience fewer and less severe depressive symptoms, suggesting that early treatment of depression would economically benefit employers.

The astounding economic costs of depression are due to a combination of direct treatment of depression, premature mortality (e.g., by suicide), and reduced productivity and absenteeism. The total annual costs of depression in the United States are estimated at US$44 billion: US$12.4 billion in direct costs of treatment (hospitals, medications, doctors' fees), US$8 billion in premature death, and US$24 billion in absenteeism and reduced productivity in the workplace. In Canada, the indirect costs of depression (premature mortality and reduced productivity) are estimated at C$2.53 billion, and represents 58% of the overall economic cost of depression. These approximations, however, underestimate the overall cost of depression because they do not include out-of-pocket family expenses, costs of minor and untreated depression, excessive hospitalization, general medical services, and diagnostic tests.

...osts of untreated depression

...ion increases the risk for both social and physical disability, ...result, increases the costs for other medical services. Nevertheless, an even greater strain on the medical system originates from the cost of undiagnosed and untreated depression. Individuals with depressive symptoms, who have not been diagnosed with a depressive disorder, utilize more medical services and attempt suicide more often than MDD diagnosed patients. In a US study, patients diagnosed with depression recovering from surgery stay on average 10 days longer in hospital than non-depressed patients. However, those individuals with untreated depressive symptoms stayed 26 days longer than non-depressed patients. In fact, individuals with untreated depression account for the majority of "high utilizers" of general medical services. Thus, diagnosing and treating these individuals should lessen the burden on the medical system.

2.3.4 **Costs of treatment**

Effective treatment of depression has been found to improve patient social functioning, lower risks of other medical illnesses, decrease lost and unproductive work days, and consequently reduce disability costs. Moreover, the use of pharmacotherapy and psychotherapy in the treatment of depression reduces the overall cost to the entire health care system. In primary care settings, the implementation of collaborative care and chronic disease management programs also has been shown to cost-effectively improve outcomes of depressed patients.

Key references

Alonso J, Angermeyer MC, Bernert S, et al. 12-month comorbidity patterns and associated factors in Europe: Results from the European Study of the Epidemiology of Mental Disorders (ESEMeD) project. *Acta Psychiatr Scand Suppl* 2004; **420**:28–37.

Badamgarav E, Weingarten SR, Henning JM, et al. Effectiveness of disease management programs in depression: a systematic review. *Am J Psychiatry* 2003; **160**:2080–90.

Cuipers P, Smit F. Excess mortality in depression: A meta-analysis of community studies. *J Affect Disord* 2002; **72**:227–36.

Kessler RC, Berglund P, Demier O, et al. The epidemiology of major depressive disorder: Results from the National Comorbidity Survey Replication (NCS-R). *JAMA* 2003; **289**:3095–105.

Parikh SV, Lam RW. Clinical guidelines for the treatment of depressive disorders. I. Definitions, prevalence and health burden. *Can J Psychiatry* 2001; **46**(Suppl 1):13S–27S.

Rost K, Smith JL, Dickinson M. The effect of improving primary care depression management on employee absenteeism and productivity. A randomized trial. *Med Care* 2004; **42**:1202–10.

Ustun TB, Ayuso-Mateos JL, Chatterji S, *et al*. Global burden of depressive disorders in the year 2000. *Br J Psychiatry* 2004; **184**:386–92.

Wang PS, Simon G, Kessler RC. The economic burden of depression and the cost-effectiveness of treatment. *Int J Methods Psychiatr Res* 2003; **12**:22–33.

Weissman MM, Bland RC, Canino GJ, *et al*. Cross-national epidemiology of major depression and bipolar disorder. *JAMA* 1996; **276**: 293–9.

Chapter 3

Pathogenesis

> **Key points**
> - There are likely multiple processes to explain the etiology and pathophysiology of depression, with the involvement of biological, psychological, and social factors.
> - Stressful life events and stress reactivity can modify genetic and biological processes to contribute to depression.
> - Endophenotypes, or genetic expressions of neural systems involved in depression, will be important in the study of the pathogenesis of depression and its treatment.

3.1 Introduction

The exact pathophysiology of major depressive disorder (MDD) remains unknown, but the etiology has always been presumed to be heterogeneous as the diagnosis of MDD is only descriptive and likely consists of a number of syndromes with related symptoms. Biological, psychological, and social factors all have influences on MDD, but new research in genetics, neuroimaging, and molecular biology has clarified some of the relationships between these broad forces, particularly in the modulation of life events on genetic and neurobiologic processes. There is increasing emphasis on endophenotypes, defined as endogenous phenotypes that are not evident to the unaided eye, that fill the gap between genes and a complex disease, to advance our classification of depressive disorders and to guide treatment selection (Figures 3.1 and 3.2). This chapter will highlight some of these recent advances.

3.2 Genetics

3.2.1 Family, twin, and adoption studies

Family studies indicate at least two or three times increased relative risk (15–25%) for MDD in first-degree relatives of MDD probands, with early age of onset and recurrent depression conferring greater risk. Adoption studies, most of them from Scandinavia, found that biological relatives of depressed adoptees were much more likely to have depression than the adoptive relatives. Twin studies, by comparing monozygotic to dizygotic twins, allow the dissection of genetic from environmental influences on disease risk. Estimates from twin studies of genetic heritability of depression range from 33 to 70%, independent of gender. The consistent results from these varied studies indicate a substantial genetic basis for MDD.

3.2.2 Linkage and association studies

Linkage analysis studies have not produced replicated results, mainly because complex disorders such as MDD are not likely to be due to abnormalities in a single gene locus. Large samples (at least 1,000 affected sibling pairs) are needed to reliably detect a locus that causes even a 30% increase in risk. Genome scanning is a powerful new tool to detect genetic associations, but results from genome scans are prone to false positive errors and need to be replicated in other large samples.

Candidate gene strategies involving association analysis to genes coding for particular elements of neurotransmitter function have been more informative (Figures 3.1 and 3.2). Particular attention has been focused on functional polymorphisms, which are variations in DNA sequences that alter the expression or functioning of gene products. Initial enthusiasm was generated for an association of MDD

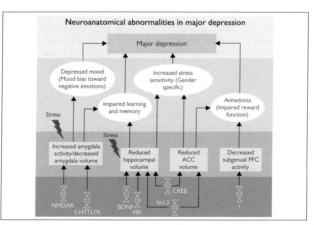

Figure 3.1 Example of how neuroanatomical abnormalities may relate to candidate genes and to key components of major depression. Not all functional directions are indicated for the sake of clarity of the figure. ACC, anterior cingulate cortex; PFC, prefrontal cortex; NMDAR, NMDA receptor; 5-HTTLPR, 5-HT (serotonin) transporter promoter region gene; BDNF, brain derived neurotrophic factor; MR, mineralocorticoid receptor; bcl-2, B-cell lymphoma-2 gene; CREB, cAMP response element binding protein. Adapted from: Hasler G, Drevets WC, Manji HK, *et al.* Discovering endophenotypes for depression. *Neuropsychopharmacol* 2004; **29**:1765–81.

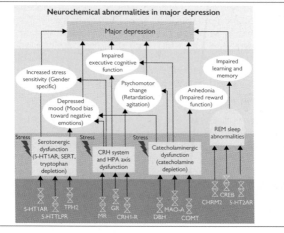

Figure 3.2 Example of how neurochemical abnormalities may relate to candidate genes and to key components of major depression. Not all functional directions are indicated for the sake of clarity of the figure. 5-HT1AR, 5-HT (serotonin) 1A receptor; SERT, serotonin transporter; CRH, corticotropin releasing hormone; HPA, hypothalamic-pituitary-adrenal axis; REM, rapid eye movement, 5-HTTLPR, 5-HT (serotonin) transporter promoter region gene; TPH-2, tryptophan hydoxylase-2; MR, mineralocorticoid receptor; GR, glucocorticoid receptor; CRH-1R, corticotropin releasing hormone-1 receptor; DBH, dopamine-beta-hydroxylase; MAO-A, monoamine oxidase-A; COMT, catechol-O-methyltransferase; CHRM2, cholinergic muscarinic-2 receptor; CREB, cAMP response element binding protein; 5-HT2AR, 5-HT (serotonin) - 2A receptor. Adapted from: Hasler G, Drevets WC, Manji HK, et al. Discovering endophenotypes for depression. *Neuropsychopharmacol* 2004; **29**:1765–81.

with the polymorphism involving the short allele of the promoter region of the serotonin transporter gene, 5-HTTLPR, and with response to SSRIs, but subsequent studies and meta-analyses have not replicated these findings. However, other evidence suggest that 5-HTTLPR polymorphisms are associated with neurotic traits and response to stressful life events, suggesting that they modify stress reactivity rather than causing MDD, per se. Other candidate genes being investigated in MDD include tryptophan hydroxylase-2, brain derived neurotrophic factor (BDNF), cAMP responsive element binding protein-1 (CREB1), and those involving the circadian clock.

3.3 Neurobiology

3.3.1 Monoamines

The monoamine hypothesis has been the foundation of neurobio-logical theories for depression for the past 50 years. Initially based upon observations of the mechanism of action of antidepressants, this hypothesis postulates that depression results from deficits in key brain areas in serotonin (5-HT) or noradrenaline synaptic neurotransmission. Antidepressants were thought to act by blocking the serotonin transporter (SERT), leading to increased availability of neurotransmitters within the synaptic cleft. However, this theory did not account for the lag time for onset of therapeutic effects of antidepressants, given that increases in synaptic neurotransmitters occur immediately with reuptake inhibitors. Tryptophan and catecholamine depletion studies also have not produced any evidence for simple deficits of neurotransmitter levels or function in MDD.

Newer models, incorporating various interdisciplinary neuroscience approaches, have extended past the synapse to focus on the importance of pre-synaptic and post-synaptic receptors and processes (Figure 3.3). For example, delayed desensitization of pre-synaptic 5-HT$_{1A}$ autoreceptors and down-regulation of post-synaptic α_2-adrenergic receptors and 5-HT$_2$ receptors have been proposed to explain the delayed response to antidepressants.

Recent molecular biology studies have shifted attention from immediate pre- or post-synaptic events to delayed post-receptor signaling pathways in the mechanism of action of antidepressants (Figure 3.3). The activation of post-synaptic receptors initiates a cascade of biochemical effects mediating signal transduction, involving G-protein coupled stimulation of cAMP or Ca^{2+} cascades. Activation of CREB results in increased expression of BDNF, which acts to promote neurogenesis (Figure 3.4), and which may account for the therapeutic effects of antidepressants (see Section 3.4).

3.3.2 **Hypothalamic-pituitary-adrenal axis**

Alterations in the hypothalamic-pituitary-adrenal (HPA) axis have long been recognized to be associated with MDD. The biological effects of stress are mediated via secretion of corticotropin releasing factor/hormone (CRF/CRH) leading to increased secretion of adrenocorticotrophic hormone (ACTH) and release of glucocorticoids. Glucocorticoids alter noradrenergic receptor sensitivity via regulation of the β-adrenoreceptor-coupled adenylate cyclase system in the brain. Chronic stress results in hypersensitivity of the HPA axis and MDD is associated with increased concentrations of CRF in the cerebrospinal fluid, increased CRF immunoreactivity and gene expression of CRF in the hypothalamic paraventricular nucleus, and down-regulation of CRF-R1 receptors in the frontal cortex. Prolonged glucocorticoid secretion has neurotoxic effects, particularly on neurogenesis in the hippocampus (Figure 3.4).

The dexamethasone suppression test in combination with the CRH-stimulation test (dex/CRH) is the most sensitive neuroendocrine measure of impaired cortisol response and HPA sensitivity. Although it has good sensitivity to detect MDD, the dex/CRH still lacks sufficient specificity (to distinguish MDD from other conditions such as schizophrenia and panic disorder) to be used as a diagnostic test. Other clinical implications of increased CRF and glucocorticoid production in MDD include the possibility that dampening the CRF response may have therapeutic effects, and several novel CRF and glucocorticoid antagonists are in early phase clinical trials as antidepressants.

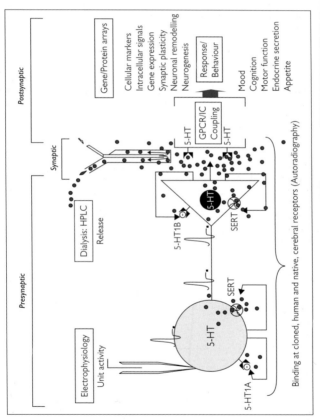

Figure 3.3 Characterization of antidepressant effects using an interdisciplinary approach. Abbreviations: 5-HT, serotonin; GPCR, G-protein coupled receptor; HPLC, high-performance liquid chromatography; IC, ion channel; SERT, serotonin transporter. Adapted from: Millan MJ. The role of monoamines in the actions of established and "novel" antidepressive agents: a critical review. *Eur J Pharmacol* 2004; **500**:371–84.

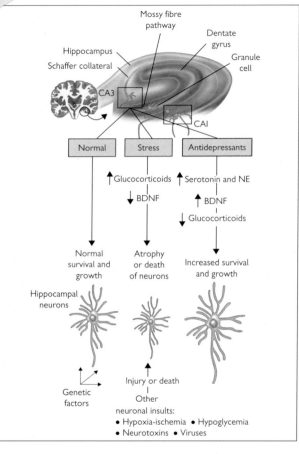

Figure 3.4 Neurogenesis hypothesis for depression and therapeutic effects of antidepressants. Abbreviations: BDNF, brain-derived neurotrophic factor; NE, norepinephrine. Adapted from: Duman RS, Heninger GR, Nestler EJ. A molecular and cellular theory of depression. *Arch Gen Psychiatry* 1997; 54:597–606.

3.3.3 **Sleep and circadian rhythms**

Sleep complaints (insomnia, hypersomnia) have long been considered cardinal features of clinical depression so it is not surprising that biological studies have focused on dysregulation of sleep in MDD. Polysomnography has been used to detect many abnormalities of sleep in MDD, and indeed offers some of the most robust biological markers in depression (Box 3.1). There remains controversy over whether depression causes sleep changes or vice versa. There is increasing evidence that sleep changes are trait markers, predate onset of depression, and predict relapse in remitted patients, thereby suggesting a pathogenic role for sleep in MDD.

Theories of sleep involve both homeostatic and circadian factors. The two-process model suggests an interactive balance between the homeostatic need for sleep, which increases with longer time awake, and a circadian propensity for sleep, which shows a circadian pattern for sleepiness and attention. Depression affects circadian rhythms such that 24-h secretion of cortisol, melatonin, and thyroid stimulating hormone is altered, with evidence for both phase shifts and decreased amplitude of rhythms. Disruptions of the circadian clock may be especially important in mood episodes associated with bipolar disorder. Circadian theories are also intimately associated with seasonal affective disorder, particularly phase-delayed circadian rhythms that are corrected by appropriately timed bright light exposure (see Chapter 7).

3.4 **Neuropsychology**

3.4.1 **Cognition and memory**

Patients with depression demonstrate a number of cognitive and memory deficits, especially in selective attention and explicit (working) memory. In addition, there are deficits in long-term storage and retrieval of declarative memory, and in executive cognitive functions such as selecting strategies and monitoring performance. Many of the cognitive problems have been associated with reduced cerebral blood flow and metabolism to dorsolateral prefrontal cortex and dorsal anterior cingulate cortex. These findings are of clinical importance for the mechanisms of cognitive-behavioural therapy for depression (see Chapter 8).

The hippocampus is critically involved in memory formation, as part of the neural circuit involved in information processing and creation of emotional and declarative memories. Hippocampal volume is decreased in patients with depression, especially with recurrent or chronic episodes or a past history of trauma. Impaired neurogenesis has been invoked to explain this finding, as increased glucocorticoid secretion from prolonged stress is particularly neurotoxic to hippocampal

> **Box 3.1 Polysomnographic abnormalities of sleep in major depressive disorder**
>
> - Early onset of rapid eye movement (REM) sleep (i.e., shortened REM latency)
> - Increased time in REM sleep
> - Increased REM density
> - Decreased slow wave sleep (SWS)
> - Shift of SWS away from the early part of the night
> - Disturbances in slow wave activity (SWA)

neurons (Figure 3.4). The neurogenesis theory also accounts for therapeutic effects of antidepressants, as these drugs activate the cAMP cascade to release BDNF and CREB, which serve to increase neurogenesis in the hippocampus.

Functional neuroimaging studies have highlighted the possibility of dysfunction in higher order organization of the brain involving specific neural circuits (Figure 3.5). These circuits link lower order subcortical functions (autonomic, regulatory) to those involving reward systems (limbic system) and higher cortical function (cognition). Network dysfunction involving limbic-cortical circuits has been shown in MDD, with changes in cortical (frontal, parietal), paralimbic (cingulate, insula) and subcortical (caudate, thalamus) activity following various types of antidepressant treatment.

In the limbic-cortical dysregulation model, alterations at various levels may produce therapeutic effects. For example, CBT may modify cortical circuits while antidepressant drugs may selectively affect circadian or other limbic circuits; the net effect of both interventions may produce the same adaptive changes in the entire system. One particularly interesting region is the subgenual cingulate, Brodmann's area Cg25, which modulates negative mood states and shows hyperactivity in depressed states while response to varied antidepressant treatment is associated with reduced activity. This is the area targeted for deep brain stimulation in preliminary studies in treatment-refractory depression (see Chapter 7).

3.4.2 **Environment and life events**

Depression often follows a major psychosocial stressor, especially with the first or second depressive episode. Adverse childhood experiences such as child abuse, loss of a parent, and inadequate social support are also common among depressed patients. Increasing evidence has determined that stress and trauma can affect biological systems of interest in depression. For example, animal studies have shown that early maternal deprivation leads to hypersensitivity of the HPA axis in adulthood, with decreased hippocampal cell proliferation similar to the reduced hippocampal volumes found in neuroimaging studies of patients with depression and childhood trauma.

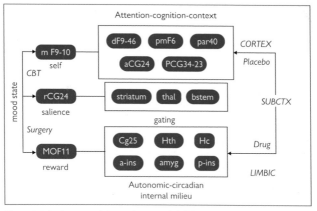

Figure 3.5 Limbic-cortical dysregulation model. Abbreviations: aCg, dorsal anterior cingulate; a-ins, anterior insula; amyg, amygdala; bstem, brainstem; Cg25, subgenual cingulate; dF, prefrontal; Hc, hippocampus; Hth, hypothalamus; mF, medial prefrontal; mOF, medial orbital frontal; par, parietal; pCg, posterior cingulate; p-ins, posterior insula; pm, premotor; rCg, rostral cingulate; thal, thalamus. Numbers are Brodmann designations. Adapted from: Mayberg HS. Modulating dysfunctional limbic-cortical circuits in depression: towards development of brain-based algorithms for diagnosis and optimised treatment. *Br Med Bull* 2003; **65**:193–207.

Twin studies have shown an interaction between genetic risk and life events for developing depression. Stressful life events had no effect on risk of developing a depression in women with the lowest genetic vulnerability, but life events had increasing effects on depression risk in those with increasing genetic loading for depression. These findings suggest that environmental events, even those that happened in the past, can alter neurobiological function for a long time. This may have implications for treatment, as studies have shown that patients with MDD and a history of early childhood trauma show better responses to psychotherapy than antidepressant monotherapy.

Key references

Armitage R. Sleep and circadian rhythms in mood disorders. *Acta Psychiatr Scand* 2007; **115**(Suppl 433):104–15.

Duman RS, Heninger GR, Nestler EJ. A molecular and cellular theory of depression. *Arch Gen Psychiatry* 1997; **54**:597–606.

Goldberg D. The aetiology of depression. *Psychol Med* 2006; **36**:1341–7.

Hasler G, Drevets WC, Manji HK, *et al*. Discovering endophenotypes for depression. *Neuropsychopharmacol* 2004; **29**:1765–81.

Kato T. Molecular genetics of bipolar disorder and depression. *Psychiatr Clin Neurosci* 2007; **61**:3–19.

Kendler KS, Kuhn JW, Vittum J, *et al*. The interaction of stressful life events and a seratonin transporter polymorphism in the prediction of episodes of major depression: a replication. *Arch Gen Psychiatry* 2005; **62**:529–35.

Levinson DF. The genetics of depression: A review. *Biol Psychiatry* 2006; **60**:84–92.

Mayberg HS. Modulating dysfunctional limbic-cortical circuits in depression: towards development of brain-based algorithms for diagnosis and optimised treatment. *Br Med Bull* 2003; **65**:193–207.

Millan MJ. The role of monoamines in the actions of established and "novel" antidepressive agents: a critical review. *Eur J Pharmacol* 2004; **500**:371–84.

Paykel E. Life events: effects and genesis. *Psychol Med* 2003; **33**:1145–8.

Taylor C, Fricker AD, Devi LA, *et al*. Mechanisms of action of antidepressants: from neurotransmitter systems to signaling pathways. *Cell Sig* 2005; **17**:549–57.

Chapter 4

Clinical features and diagnosis

Key points
• Depression is associated with a number of physical, emotional, and cognitive symptoms.
• The differential diagnosis of depression includes bereavement, bipolar disorder, and other medical or substance-induced conditions.
• Sub-typing of major depressive disorder has implications for treatment choice and selection.

4.1 Clinical features

4.1.1 Overview

Depression is associated with many different types of symptoms that can result in a variable presentation in any given person. The features of depression can be physical (sleep, energy, appetite, libido), emotional (low mood, anxiety, crying) or cognitive (guilt, pessimism, suicidal thoughts). Table 4.1 presents a common mnemonic for depressive symptoms.

Table 4.1 SIGECAPS mnemonic for the clinical features of depression	
Depressive symptom (SIGECAPS)	**Presentation**
Sleep	• Insomnia or hypersomnia (atypical)
Interest/pleasure	• Decreased (anhedonia)
Guilt	• Increased, irrational/delusional thoughts
Energy	• Decreased (fatigue)
Concentration	• Decreased; indecisive and distractible
Appetite	• Decreased or increased (atypical)
Psychomotor activity	• Agitation or retardation
Suicide	• Thoughts, plans, attempts

i.2 **Symptoms**

Low mood. While depressed people describe feelings of low mood, the emotional misery experienced during a depression is qualitatively different from normal periods of sadness or grief that everyone experiences. Some have crying spells, or feel like crying, while others describe a complete lack of emotional response.

Interest/pleasure. Loss of interest and pleasure in activities or social interactions that previously were pleasurable is another cardinal feature of depression. Anhedonia also may show as indifference or boredom, and can be present even when the person does not endorse low mood. Loss of sexual interest, desire, or functioning is also common, which can lead to difficulty in intimate relationships and marital conflict.

Sleep. Most depressed patients experience sleeping difficulties. The classic presentation is waking from sleep early in the morning and being unable to fall asleep again (terminal insomnia), but restless sleep and frequent waking during the night (middle insomnia) is also common. Difficulty falling asleep at the beginning of the night (early or initial insomnia) is usually seen when anxiety also is present. In contrast, hypersomnia or oversleeping also can be a symptom of depression.

Energy. Low energy and fatigue are frequent complaints in depression, as is difficulty in getting started or initiating tasks. The fatigue experienced can be physical or mental, and may be associated with poor sleep and appetite. In severe cases, routine activities such as daily hygiene, grooming, or eating may be impaired. An extreme form of fatigue is "leaden paralysis," in which patients describe a feeling like their limbs are made of lead, or that they are walking through water.

Guilt. Feelings of worthlessness and guilt can often consume an individual's thoughts during a depressive episode. Depressed patients may misinterpret trivial daily events and take responsibility for negative events out of their control; these can sometimes be of delusional proportion. Excessive worry and anxiety can accompany and exacerbate guilt.

Concentration. Difficulty with concentration and decision making is often experienced in depression. Memory complaints are usually due to problems with attention and distractibility. In elderly patients, the cognitive complaints may be misdiagnosed as early dementia. The concentration and memory problems can greatly impair work function, especially in "white collar" workers.

Appetite/weight. Loss of appetite, taste, and enjoyment in eating can lead to significant weight loss and some patients may need to "force" themselves to eat. However, other patients may crave carbohydrates and sweets when depressed, or self-treat by "comfort" eating. Overeating, accompanied by decreased activity and exercise, can lead to weight gain and metabolic syndrome. Changes in weight may also impact on self-image and self-esteem.

Psychomotor activity. Psychomotor changes, which are subjective changes in motor function without objective abnormalities on testing, are commonly seen in depression. Psychomotor retardation consists of slowing (slowed body movements, lack of facial expression, long latency of speech response) which, at its extreme, can manifest as mute or catatonic presentations. Anxiety can also present as psychomotor agitation (talking quickly, pacing, restlessness, inability to sit still). Racing thoughts may be a symptom of mania, but can also indicate anxiety.

Suicide. Some type of suicidal ideation, ranging from fleeting thoughts of wishing everything would end to elaborate plans for suicide, is present in nearly two-thirds of people with depression. Even when suicidal thoughts are serious, depressed patients often lack the energy and motivation to attempt suicide. However, suicide remains a significant issue as 10–15% of hospitalized depressed individuals eventually die by suicide. A period of high risk for suicide is during initial treatment, when energy and motivation may improve before the cognitive symptoms (e.g., hopelessness), making it possible for suicidal patients to act on their thoughts and plans.

Other symptoms. Anxiety, with its many subjective and physical manifestations, is very common in depression. Increased irritability and mood swings, outbursts of anger or sadness, and frustration and irritation over minor matters also are frequently seen. Diurnal variation of mood, with morning worsening, may be present. A depression often assaults self-esteem and self-worth, with thoughts of worthlessness accompanying hopelessness. Depression also is associated with increased frequency and magnification of physical pain, including headaches, backaches, and other chronic painful conditions.

4.2 **Classification and diagnosis of depression**

4.2.1 **Classification of depression**

The DSM-IV-TR outlines three major sub-classifications for depression: major depressive disorder (MDD), dysthymia, and depressive disorder not otherwise specified (NOS). Figure 4.1 outlines a simple algorithm to distinguish these depressive disorders from bipolar disorder.

4.2.2 **Major depressive disorder**

Major depressive disorder (MDD) is characterized by the presence of one or more major depressive episodes (Box 4.1). The diagnostic criteria require a threshold number of symptoms that m⌊

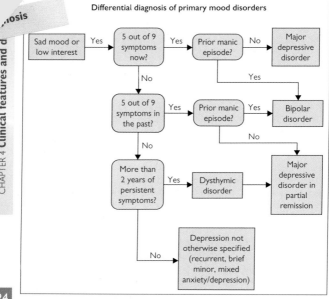

Figure 4.1 Differential diagnosis of depression. Adapted from: US Department of Health and Human Services. Depression in Primary Care, Volume 1. Detection and Diagnosis. AHCPR Publication No. 93-0550, Agency for Health Care Policy and Research, Rockville, MD 1993, p. 20.

present much of the time, most days, for at least 2 weeks, although the duration is usually much longer by the time help is sought. The symptoms also must significantly impair function. Finally, bereavement and other causes of depressive symptoms must be excluded.

MDD is identified as either single episode or recurrent, with the latter consisting of two or more major depressive episodes with a remission interval of at least 2 months. MDD can also be "sub-typed" according to several specifiers and by severity; these can be used to differentiate presentations of depression that have implications for recognition (distinctive symptoms or pattern), prognosis, or treatment selection.

Box 4.1 DSM-IV-TR criteria for the diagnosis of a major depressive episode

A. Five (or more) of the following symptoms have been present during the same 2-week period and represent a change from previous functioning; at least one of the symptoms is either (1) depressed mood or (2) loss of interest or pleasure.

1. Depressed mood most of the day or nearly every day, as indicated by either a subjective report (e.g., feels sad or empty) or observation made by others (e.g., appears tearful). Note: In children and adolescents, can be irritable mood.

2. Markedly diminished interest or pleasure in all, or almost all, activities most of the day, nearly every day (as indicated by either subjective account or observation made by others).

3. Significant weight loss when not dieting or weight gain (e.g., a change of more than 5% of body weight in a month), or decrease or increase in appetite nearly every day. Note: In children, consider failure to make expected weight gains.

4. Insomnia or hypersomnia nearly every day.

5. Psychomotor agitation or retardation nearly every day (observable by others, not merely subjective feelings of restlessness or being slowed down).

6. Fatigue or loss of energy nearly every day.

7. Feelings of worthlessness or excessive or inappropriate guilt (which may be delusional) nearly every day (not merely self-reproach or guilt about being sick).

8. Diminished ability to think or concentrate, or indecisiveness, nearly every day (either by subjective account or as observed by others).

9. Recurrent thoughts of death (not just fear of dying), recurrent suicidal ideation without a specific plan, or a suicide attempt or a specific plan for committing suicide.

B. The symptoms do not meet criteria for a mixed episode.

C. The symptoms cause clinically significant distress or impairment in social, occupational, or other important areas of functioning.

D. The symptoms are not due to the direct physiological effects of a substance (e.g., a drug of abuse, a medication) or a general medical condition (e.g., hypothyroidism).

E. The symptoms are not better accounted for by bereavement.

4.2.3 **Dysthymia**

Dysthymia is a chronic, low grade mood disorder during which the full criteria for a major depressive episode are not met (Box 4.2). Dysthymic symptoms develop slowly, often unrecognized by the individual, and persist for a minimum of 2 years (median 5 years). Individuals with dysthymia often develop episodes of major depression (termed "double depressions"), which may prompt them to seek treatment.

Box 4.2 **DSM-IV-TR diagnostic criteria for dysthymia**

A. Depressed mood for most of the day, for more days than not, as indicated either by a subjective account or observation by others, for at least 2 years. Note: In children and adolescents, mood can be irritable and duration must be at least 1 year.

B. Presence, while depressed, of two (or more) of the following:
   1. poor appetite or overeating
   2. insomnia or hypersomnia
   3. low energy or fatigue
   4. low self-esteem
   5. poor concentration or difficulty making decisions
   6. feelings of hopelessness.

C. During the 2-year period (1 year for children or adolescents) of the disturbance, the person has never been without the symptoms in criteria A and B for more than 2 months at a time.

D. No major depressive episode was present during the first 2 years of the disturbance (1 year for children and adolescents); that is, the disturbance is not better accounted for by chronic major depressive disorder, or major depressive disorder, in partial remission.

Note: There may have been a previous major depressive episode provided there was a full remission (no significant signs or symptoms for 2 months) before development of the dysthymic disorder. In addition, after the initial 2 years (1 year in children or adolescents) of dysthymic disorder, there may be superimposed episodes of major depressive disorder, in which case both diagnoses may be given when the criteria are met for a major depressive episode.

E. There has never been a manic episode, a mixed episode, or a hypomanic episode, and criteria have never been met for cyclothymic disorder.

F. The disturbance does not occur exclusively during the course of a chronic psychotic disorder, such as schizophrenia or delusional disorder.

G. The symptoms are not due to the direct physiological effects of a substance (e.g., a drug of abuse, a medication) or a general medical condition (e.g., hypothyroidism).

H. The symptoms cause clinically significant distress or impairment in social, occupational, or other important areas of functioning.

> **Box 4.3 DSM-IV-TR examples of depressive disorder not otherwise specified**
>
> - **Premenstrual dysphoric disorder**: In most menstrual cycles during the past year, symptoms regularly occurred during the last week of the luteal phase and remitted within a few days of the onset of menses.
> - **Minor depressive disorder**: Episodes of at least 2 weeks of depressive symptoms but with fewer than the five items required for MDD.
> - **Recurrent brief depressive disorder**: Depressive episodes lasting from 2 days up to 2 weeks, occurring at least once a month for 12 months and not associated with the menstrual cycle.
> - **Post-psychotic depressive disorder of schizophrenia**: An MDE that occurs during the residual phase of schizophrenia.
> - **An MDE superimposed on the following**: Delusional disorder, psychotic disorder not otherwise specified, or the active phase of schizophrenia.
> - **Situations in which the physician has concluded** that a depressive disorder is present but is unable to determine whether it is primary, due to a general medical condition, or substance-induced.

4.2.4 **Depressive disorder not otherwise specified**

Depressive disorder NOS involves other depressive conditions that do not meet criteria for the main depressive disorders (Box 4.3). Some of these conditions, such as minor depression and recurrent brief depression, are under study for inclusion in future diagnostic classifications.

4.2 **Types of depression**

4.3.1 **Specifiers of major depressive disorder**

Several specifiers (sub-types) of MDD have been established based on clinical features and patterns of depressive episodes. These DSM-IV-TR depressive specifiers sub-classify depression with the intent to improve treatment selection and predict prognosis. Table 4.2 outlines the depressive specifiers along with their key features.

Although not identified as a specifier of depression within DSM-IV-TR, "anxious depression" is a term that describes a proportion of depressed patients (60–90%) that experience symptoms of anxiety (e.g., excessive worry, tension, and somatic symptoms related to anxiety). Individuals with anxious depression experience greater functional and psychosocial disability with a greater risk of suicide and a poorer prognosis, as compared to those with low anxiety.

Table 4.2 **DSM-IV-TR sub-types and specifiers of MDD**

Sub-type	DSM-IV-TR specifier	Key features
Melancholic depression	With melancholic features	Nonreactive mood, anhedonia, weight loss, guilt, psychomotor retardation or agitation, morning worsening of mood, early morning awakening
Atypical depression	With atypical features	Reactive mood, over-sleeping, over-eating, leaden paralysis, interpersonal rejection sensitivity
Psychotic (delusional) depression	With psychotic features	Hallucinations or delusions
Catatonic depression	With catatonic features	Catalepsy (waxy flexibility), catatonic excitement, negativism or mutism, mannerisms or stereotypies, echolalia or echopraxia. (uncommon in clinical practice)
Chronic depression	Chronic pattern	Two years or more with full criteria for MDE
Seasonal affective disorder (SAD)	Seasonal pattern	Regular onset and remission of depressive episodes during a particular season (usually fall/winter onset)
Postpartum depression (PPD)	Postpartum pattern	Onset of depressive episode within 4 weeks postpartum

4.3.2 Severity

Both the DSM-IV-TR and the ICD-10 categorize three separate levels of severity for MDD: mild, moderate, and severe (Table 4.3). The DSM-IV-TR distinguishes the severity based on the effect the depression has on the social/occupational roles and responsibilities of the individual and the presence of psychotic features. The ICD-10, on the other hand, differentiates the severity of depression based on the number and type of symptoms present in the depressed individual. The use of validated depression rating scales is recommended for assessing severity (see Chapter 5 and Appendix).

Severity of depression may influence treatment choices. For example, psychotherapy is as effective as pharmacotherapy for mild to moderate depression, but severe depression shows better response to combination treatment. Emerging evidence also suggests that some antidepressants may be more effective than others for severe depression (see Chapter 6).

Table 4.3 Depression severity criteria		
Depression severity	**DSM-IV-TR criteria**	**ICD-10 criteria**
Mild	1 Depressed mood or loss of interest/pleasure + four other depressive symptoms 2 Minor social/occupation impairment	1 Two typical symptoms 2 Two other core symptoms
Moderate	1 Depressed mood or loss of interest/pleasure + four or more other depressive symptoms 2 Variable social/occupational impairment	1 Two typical symptoms 2 Three or more other core symptoms
Severe	1 Depressed mood or loss of interest/pleasure + four or more other depressive symptoms 2 Major social/occupational impairment—or with psychotic features	1 Three typical symptoms 2 Four or more other core symptoms Also subtyped as with or without psychotic symptoms

4.2 Differential diagnosis

4.4.1 Bereavement

Bereavement or grief over loss of relationships can share similar symptoms with a major depressive episode. Severity and duration of symptoms and their impact on psychosocial function can help distinguish between grief and MDD (Table 4.4).

4.4.2 Mood disorder due to a general medical condition

Depressive symptoms can result from the direct physiological effects of a specific pre-existing medical condition. Conversely, the physical symptoms of a primary medical illness may obscure the diagnosis of a comorbid MDD (see Chapter 9). The Hospital Anxiety and Depression Scale (HADS) is a useful screening tool for medically ill patients in that it uses questions that focus on cognitive symptoms rather than somatic ones. MDD is prevalent in numerous chronic illnesses (Table 4.5), but may be particularly common in diabetes, cardiovascular disease (e.g., post-myocardial infarction), thyroid disease, and neurological disorders (e.g., Parkinson's disease, multiple sclerosis).

4.4.3 Substance-induced mood disorder

Side effects of drugs (whether prescribed or illicit) can also lead to depressive symptoms, so substance-induced mood disorders must be considered in the differential diagnosis of MDD (Box 4.4). Evidence from the history, physical examination, or laboratory findings are used to establish whether abuse, dependence, intoxication, or withdrawal states are physiologically inducing a depressive episode. While substance-induced depressive symptoms usually resolve with discontinuation of the substance, some intense forms of withdrawal can last over a month.

Table 4.4 Features distinguishing between bereavement and a major depressive episode

Feature	Bereavement	Major depressive episode
Time course	Less than 2 months	More than 2 months
Feelings of worthlessness	Absent	Present
Suicidal ideas	Absent	Common
Delusions of guilt, etc.	Absent	Possible
Psychomotor changes	Mild agitation	Marked slowing
Functional impairment	Mild	Marked to severe

Table 4.5 General medical conditions associated with depressive symptoms

Neurological disorders
- Alzheimer's disease
- Cerebrovascular disease
- Cerebral neoplasms
- Cerebral trauma
- CNS infections
- Dementia
- Epilepsy
- Extrapyramidal diseases
- Huntington's disease
- Hydrocephalus
- Migraine
- Multiple Sclerosis
- Narcolepsy
- Parkinson's disease
- Progressive supranuclear palsy
- Sleep apnea
- Wilson's disease

Systemic disorders
- Viral and bacterial infections

Inflammatory disorders
- Rheumatoid arthritis
- Sjogren's syndrome
- Systemic lupus erythematosis
- Temporal arteritis

Endocrine disorders
- Adrenal
  1. Cushing's
  2. Addison's
  3. Hyperaldosteronism
- Menses related
- Parathyroid disorders
- Thyroid disorders
- Vitamin deficiencies
  1. B12/Folate
  2. Vitamin C
  3. Niacin
  4. Thiamine

Other disorders
- Acquired immune deficiency syndrome (AIDS)
- Cancer
- Cardiopulmonary disease
- Klinefelter's syndrome
- Myocardial infarction
- Porphyrias
- Postoperative states
- Renal disease and uremia
- Systemic neoplasms

4.4.4 Bipolar disorder

A history of mania or hypomania signifies a bipolar disorder, but since (1) bipolar disorder often starts with a depressive episode, and (2) bipolar patients spend more time in depressive episodes than in mania/hypomania, it is important to carefully rule out bipolarity when diagnosing MDD. In fact, 5–10% of individuals that experience a major depressive episode will have a manic or hypomanic episode in their lifetime. Depressive symptoms that suggest bipolarity include racing thoughts, psychotic symptoms, atypical features (hypersomnia, overeating), early age of onset, and recurrent episodes. Bipolar II (with hypomania) disorder is especially difficult to recognize because patients do not recognize hypomania as abnormal—they may simply perceive it as feeling good. Collateral information from a spouse, close friend, or family member is often essential to making this diagnosis. Validated screening questionnaires, such as the Mood Disorders Questionnaire, can also be helpful for identifying hypomania.

> **Box 4.4 Common drugs of abuse resulting in substance-induced mood disorders**
>
> - Alcohol
> - Amphetamines
> - Anxiolytics
> - Cocaine
> - Hallucinogens
> - Hypnotics
> - Inhalants
> - Opioids
> - Phencycline
> - Sedatives

Key references

American Psychiatric Association. *Diagnostic and Statistical Manual of Mental Disorders*, 4th edition, text revision. Washington, DC: American Psychiatric Press, 2000.

American Psychiatric Association. Practice guideline for the assessment and treatment of patients with suicidal behaviours. *Am J Psychiatry* 2003; **160**(Suppl 11):1–60.

Evans DL, Charney DS, Lewis L, *et al.* Mood disorders in the medically ill: Scientific review and recommendations. *Biol Psychiatry* 2005; **58**(3):175–89.

Hirschfeld RM, Williams JB, Spitzer RL, *et al.* Development and validation of a screening instrument for bipolar spectrum disorder: the Mood Disorder Questionnaire. *Am J Psychiatry* 2000; **157**:1873–5.

Reesal RT, Lam RW. Clinical guidelines for the treatment of depressive disorders. II. Principles of management. *Can J Psychiatry* 2001; **46**(Suppl 1): 21S–28S.

World Health Organization. International Statistical Classification of Diseases and Health Related Problems (ICD-10) 2nd edition. Geneva, CH: World Health Organization, 2005.

Zigmond AS, Snaith RP. The hospital anxiety and depression scale. *Acta Psychiatr Scand* 1983; **67**:361–70.

Chapter 5

Clinical management

> **Key points**
> - Clinical management of depression includes screening, assessment, developing a therapeutic alliance, selecting treatment(s), monitoring, and follow-up.
> - The treatment of depression has two phases: the acute phase to achieve full remission of symptoms, and the maintenance phase to prevent relapse and recurrence.
> - Self-management is an important component of disease management programs for depression.

5.1 Introduction

Clinical management for patients with depression involves following general principles of care: careful assessment, developing a therapeutic alliance, selecting evidence-based treatments, monitoring outcomes, and following up appropriately. Understanding that treatment of depression has two phases, acute and maintenance, will ensure that patients not only get well, but also stay well. For many patients, depression can be considered a recurrent or chronic illness, so following principles of chronic disease management (CDM) will also help improve outcomes. CDM, which is widely used for medical conditions such as diabetes and arthritis, includes elements of screening, self-management, monitoring, collaborative care, and rehabilitation.

33

5.2 Assessment

5.1.1 Screening

Depression is not easily diagnosed, especially in primary care settings, because often the presenting complaint is physical (e.g., body aches, fatigue, insomnia, etc.). Some depressed individuals are unaware of sad mood, or are feeling lack of emotion. In these cases, asking about loss of interest or pleasure can be diagnostic. People with high risk factors should be screened for a depressive illness (Box 5.1).

Box 5.1 Patients with the following factors are at high risk for MDD and should be screened

- Chronic pain
- Chronic physical illness (diabetes, heart disease, etc.)
- Unexplained somatic symptoms
- Frequent visits to primary care setting
- Postpartum state
- Recent psychosocial stressors

If these risk factors are present, a two-question "quick screening tool" can be used. An answer of "Yes" to either question indicates that a more detailed assessment is required.

1. In the last month, have you been bothered by little interest or pleasure in doing things?
2. In the last month, have you been feeling down, depressed, or hopeless?

5.1.2 Diagnostic tools

There are no specific laboratory tests to guide diagnosis, so the diagnostic interview remains the "gold standard" in psychiatry. However, semi-structured interviews and questionnaires can help a busy clinician to more efficiently establish the diagnostic criteria and to ensure a complete functional inquiry. Examples of such instruments include the PRIME-MD (useful in primary care settings), the Structured Clinical Interview for DSM-IV-TR (SCID, used in many psychiatric research studies), and the Mini International Neuropsychiatric Interview (MINI, more convenient and clinician-friendly; available for free download at www.medical-outcomes.com).

5.1.3 Suicide assessment

Suicide is one of the most tragic consequences of depression. It is difficult to predict suicide risk beyond very short time periods. Table 5.1 lists risk factors for suicide based on episode characteristics and demographics, but these give only a general sense of suicide potential. For any given patient, different factors will be important.

In the assessment of suicidality, attention must be given to social supports, potential methods, lethality of previous attempts and plans, and personality traits such as impulsivity. The period of initiating treatment is a time of higher suicide risk, in part because symptoms tend to be most severe before seeking help, the patient may be having initial side effects (such as anxiety or agitation) that can worsen suicidality, and patients may improve in physical symptoms (e.g., energy) before cognitive symptoms (e.g., hopelessness) and thereby be more likely to act on suicidal impulses.

Table 5.1 Risk factors for suicide	
Related to episode	**Related to demographics**
• Current suicidal plans • Prior attempts • Severe depression • Hopelessness and guilt • Inpatient or recently discharged • Bipolarity (especially Bipolar II) • Mixed state (with agitation), dysphoric mania • Psychotic features • Comorbidity (anxiety, substance abuse, serious medical conditions)	• Male • Adolescent or elderly • Early onset of mood disorder • Personality disorder (especially Cluster B) • Family history of suicide • Adverse childhood experiences (trauma, illness, parental loss) • Adverse life circumstances (unemployment, social isolation) • Recent psychosocial stressor • Lack of supports

Management of suicidal ideation includes minimizing available methods for suicide (removing guns, prescribing small amounts of medication), substituting an activity (going for a walk, doing relaxation exercises, etc.), keeping a list of reasons for living, and making contingency plans (e.g., contacting a crisis telephone line, calling a friend, going to the emergency room). Although contracts against suicide (verbal or written) are widely used by clinicians, they have not been shown to be effective in the management of suicidal patients. Documentation of suicidality and management plans, however, is very important. Some patients with acute and severe suicidality will require civil committal to hospital under regional mental health legislation.

5.1.4 Monitoring outcomes

Outcome is best monitored by the use of validated symptom rating scales, which are psychiatry's version of laboratory tests. The benefits of rating scales include comprehensive assessment of symptoms, reliable measurement of treatment effects, ensuring full remission is achieved, and aiding patient education and self-management.

Rating scales can be clinician-administered or patient-rated. Self-rated scales can help improve efficiency for busy clinicians because they can be completed at home or in the waiting room, and can also be used by patients to monitor their own mood states. The most widely used clinician-based depression scales are the Hamilton Depression (HAM-D) Rating Scale and the Montgomery–Asberg Depression Rating Scale (MADRS). Commonly used patient-rated scales include the Beck Depression Inventory II, the Hospital Anxiety and Depression Scale (HADS), the Patient Health Questionnaire (PHQ-9, specifically developed for primary care settings) the Quick Inventory for Depressive Symptomatology (QIDS-SR, used in the STAR*D study, see Chapter 9) and the Zung Self-rating Depression Scale. Some of these rating scales are found in the Appendix.

response is often defined as 50% or greater reduction from ... ...e in depression rating scale scores, which indicates substantial ...nd meaningful improvement. However, despite this clinical improvement, patients may be left with residual symptoms of depression. Many studies have shown that residual symptoms are associated with poorer outcomes, including higher risks of relapse, chronicity, suicide, and poor social and occupational function. Therefore, the target for treatment should be remission of symptoms, which is defined as a rating scale score within the normal, not depressed range (e.g., MADRS score ≤10, HAM-D score ≤7, QIDS-SR ≤5).

5.2 Phases of treatment

The treatment of depression can be divided into two phases, acute and maintenance, with different goals and activities (Table 5.2). For most patients, successful management of depression takes at least 1 year, but for some patients, treatment will need to continue for 2 years or more.

In the acute phase, symptom remission is often considered the target for treatment. However, restoration of function is more meaningful to patients and should be the ultimate goal of treatment. Full recovery of function, however, may take longer to achieve, and is unlikely to happen unless symptom remission occurs.

Table 5.2 Phases of treatment for depression

Phase	Duration	Goals	Activities
Acute	• 8–12 weeks	• Remission of symptoms • Improvement in social and occupational function	• Establish a therapeutic alliance • Educate and aid self-management • Choose treatment(s) • Manage side effects • Follow up and monitor outcomes
Maintenance	• 6–24 months or longer	• Return to baseline social and occupational function • Prevention of relapse and recurrence	• Educate and aid self-management • Manage side effects • Rehabilitate work and social function • Monitor for recurrence

Box 5.2 Maintenance pharmacotherapy recommendations

1. All patients should continue pharmacotherapy for at least 6 months following remission of symptoms.
2. Patients with the following risk factors should be maintained on pharmacotherapy for at least 2 years (up to lifetime for some patients):
   - Severe episodes
   - Chronic episodes
   - Comorbid episodes
   - Difficult-to-treat episodes
   - Frequent episodes
   - Older age

Maintenance treatment is particularly important for pharmacotherapy, as relapse or recurrence is likely to occur if medications are stopped too soon. Meta-analyses have shown that maintenance antidepressants can reduce relapse rates to 10–20% compared to 50% or higher rates with placebo. For uncomplicated depressive episodes, maintenance of 6 months appears sufficient, but 2 or more years is recommended when risk factors are present (Box 5.2).

5.3 Clinical management

5.3.1 Choice of treatment

Selecting a treatment must include an evaluation of severity of illness, availability of resources, and patient preference. For depressions of mild to moderate severity, evidence-based psychotherapies are as effective as pharmacotherapy. There is little evidence that combining pharmacotherapy and psychotherapy for initial treatment is superior to either treatment alone for uncomplicated depressions. Therefore, combination treatment should be considered when the depression is severe, comorbid with other conditions, or there is inadequate response to monotherapy.

5.3.2 Optimizing adherence

Methods for enhancing adherence to pharmacotherapy include giving some simple instructions to every patient starting on medications (Box 5.3).

> ### Box 5.3 Simple messages to give to patients to improve adherence to pharmacotherapy
>
> - Antidepressants are not addictive.
> - Take your medications every day, as prescribed.
> - It may take 2 or 3 weeks before you start feeling better.
> - Mild side effects are expected, but should get better with time.
> - Call me before you stop the medication.

5.3.3 Collaborative care

Collaborative care refers to patients receiving depression care from more than one provider. In most cases, this will be a physician prescribing medications and another practitioner (nurse, psychologist, etc.) providing psychotherapy. In some primary care settings, patients may have access to a care manager who provides education, support and, sometimes, brief psychotherapy. Care management by telephone has been shown to have similar effects to face-to-face meetings, and is more convenient and cost-effective to implement across clinical settings. Studies have shown that these collaborative care programs, including telephone care management, lead to improved outcomes, with a favorable cost-offset.

In situations where another health professional is providing psychotherapy, it is still important for the primary physician to monitor outcomes, so that other treatments (e.g., pharmacotherapy) can be applied if improvement is not seen after an appropriate follow-up period.

5.3.4 Follow-up

Health service studies show that, in primary care settings, an average of three office visits take place in the first 6 months after a diagnosis of depression is made. This is not considered adequate follow-up for depression management, and may be a factor in less than optimal outcomes associated with depression treatment in "usual care." It is especially important to monitor more frequently in the first weeks of treatment, as this is a period with higher suicide risk, challenges to adherence, and potential clinical worsening. Follow-up visits may be brief, but the suggested frequency is weekly for the first 4 weeks, then monthly for 6 months, then every 3 months, as needed.

5.3.5 Patient education and self-management

Self-management is an integral focus for CDM approaches. At its simplest, self-management includes educating patients about the illness and its treatment. At more complex levels, it includes active involvement of patients in their own recovery, using techniques taken primarily from CBT and recovery models. Patient self-help and support groups are also important resources that are often available locally.

Table 5.3 Resources for self-management

Recommended Books

- *Antidepressant Skills Workbook* by Dan Bilsker, PhD, and Randy J. Paterson, PhD. BC Mental Health and Addiction Services, 2006; Available for free download at: www.CARMHA.ca/publications
- *The Feeling Good Handbook* by Dr. David D. Burns. New York: Penguin Books, 1999.
- *Mind Over Mood* by David Greenberger, PhD, and Christine Padesky, PhD. New York: Guildford Press, 1995.

Recommended Internet sites	
www.canmat.org	Canadian Network for Mood and Anxiety Treatments (guidelines, public info)
www.heretohelp.org	BC Partners for Mental Health, Canada (public info)
www.mentalhealth.com	Internet Mental Health, Canada (public info)
www.depression.org.uk	Stress, Anxiety and Depression (STRAND), UK (public info)
www.nimh.org	National Institute of Mental Health, USA
www.primarycare.org	MacArthur Foundation Primary Care Initiative, USA
www.bluepages.anu.edu.au	Blue Pages, Australia (public info)
www.DepNet.com	Internet community support site, Australia, Canada, Denmark, Korea, Singapore, South Africa

Bibliotherapy, including workbooks for patients (Table 5.3), is effective as monotherapy for patients with mild depression, and can be used as adjunctive treatment for more severe cases. The Internet is becoming increasingly important as a source of information for self-management of medical conditions. Table 5.3 lists some resources for self-management.

Key references

Badamgarav E, Weingarten SR, Henning JM, et al. Effectiveness of disease management programs in depression: a systematic review. *Am J Psychiatry* 2003; **160**:2080–90.

Gilbody S, Whitty P, Grimshaw J, Thomas R. Educational and organizational interventions to improve the management of depression in primary care: a systematic review. *JAMA* 2003; **289**:3145–51.

Lam RW, Michalak EE, Swinson RP. *Assessment Scales in Depression, Mania and Anxiety*. London: Taylor and Francis, 2005.

Reesal RT, Lam RW, CANMAT Depression Work Group. Clinical guidelines for the treatment of depressive disorders. II. Principles of management. *Can J Psychiatry* 2001; **46**(Suppl 1): 21S–28S.

Trivedi MH, Rush AJ, Wisniewski SR, *et al.* Evaluation of outcomes with citalopram for depression using measurement-based care in STAR*D: implications for clinical practice. *Am J Psychiatry* 2006; **163**:28–40.

Von Korff M, Glasgow RE, Sharpe M. ABC of psychological medicine: organizing care for chronic illness. *BMJ* 2002; **325**:92–94.

Young AS, Alpers DH, Norland CC, *et al.* The quality of care for depressive and anxiety disorders in the United States. *Arch Gen Psychiatry* 2001; **58**:55–61.

Chapter 6

Pharmacotherapy

> ### Key points
>
> - The newer antidepressants (SSRIs, ASRI, SNRIs, other receptor agents) are first-line medications due to improved safety and tolerability over first-generation medications (TCAs, MAOIs).
> - Selection of an antidepressant must take into account efficacy, depression subtype, safety, side effect profile, simplicity of use, comorbid conditions, concurrent medications, and cost.
> - Switching antidepressants must take into account side effects, discontinuation effects, potential drug interactions, and rapidity of switch.

6.1 Selecting an antidepressant

There are only small differences in efficacy among the antidepressants, so efficacy alone cannot be the only factor in selecting a medication. Other factors that must be considered include safety, tolerability, simplicity of use, comorbid conditions, potential drug interactions, subtype of depression, and cost. For most clinical situations, there is usually no single medication of choice, and side effect profile tends to be the factor given highest priority by clinicians in selecting an antidepressant. All of the newer, second-generation antidepressants are considered first-line medications because they are safer and better tolerated than the older, first-generation tricyclic antidepressants (TCAs) and monoamine oxidase inhibitors (MAOIs).

6.2 Comparative efficacy

There are many antidepressants with proven efficacy against placebo, but there is little information on differences in efficacy among the available antidepressants. A major methodological problem is that it is much more difficult to power studies to detect the smaller but still clinically relevant differences between two active drugs than to find the larger differences between drug and placebo. Statistical calculations show that a randomized controlled trial (RCT) requires over 400 patients in each group to demonstrate a 10% difference in efficacy between two active drugs; there are no RCTs that large for any

41

psychiatric condition. Consequently, there is increasing use of meta-analysis, a statistical technique to combine results from studies involving smaller samples, to investigate comparative efficacy. There are several limitations to this approach. For example, establishing equivalent doses among the different medications is difficult. Some of these meta-analyses group together classes of medications (e.g., selective serotonin reuptake inhibitors—SSRIs), but this may not be appropriate since it is not clear whether all these medications, even within the SSRI class, have the same efficacy profile (e.g., non-response to one SSRI does not predict non-response to another, and vice versa).

With these limitations in mind, there is reasonable evidence from meta-analyses that venlafaxine, particularly at higher doses, has a greater likelihood of producing remission than SSRI agents. Meta-analyses have consistently shown 7–10% superiority in remission rates for venlafaxine compared to SSRIs (primarily fluoxetine), leading to a number needed to treat (NNT) of 10–12 (i.e., need to treat 10 patients with venlafaxine to achieve 1 more remission than treating with an SSRI; or, for every 100 patients treated with venlafaxine, 10 more will go into remission than with SSRIs). The superiority of venlafaxine has not been shown against other agents such as bupropion, duloxetine, escitalopram or mirtazapine. Meta-analyses also show that escitalopram is consistently superior to citalopram and other SSRIs, with an effect size and NNT similar to that of venlafaxine/SSRI comparisons (i.e., for every 100 patients treated with escitalopram, 11 more will go into remission than with citalopram).

In the subpopulation of patients with more severe illness (and its proxy, hospitalized patient samples), the TCA clomipramine was found to be superior to SSRIs and moclobemide. Meta-analyses show that the clomipramine results do not extend to other TCAs such as amitriptyline and imipramine. In prospective head-to-head RCTs, escitalopram also shows superiority to citalopram and paroxetine in severe depression.

Given that anxiety and depression are frequently comorbid, antidepressants with broad spectrum efficacy, that is, those that are effective for both depressive and anxiety disorders, carry an advantage for clinical use. The SSRIs, escitalopram, and venlafaxine have good evidence for efficacy in a number of anxiety disorders.

6.3 Safety

The newer antidepressants have superseded TCAs and MAOIs in clinical use because of their superior tolerability and safety profile. The absence of cardiovascular side effects makes SSRIs and other new agents much safer in both overdose and in potential drug interactions. However, there has been increasing public and professional attention to the possibility that antidepressants, particularly SSRIs and other second-generation agents, may worsen suicidality, defined as suicidal ideation and attempts. While this issue was first raised in the pediatric trials (see Chapter 9), suicidality with antidepressants has also been queried in adult populations.

Reviews of meta-analyses and large-sample naturalistic database studies, however, do not show evidence of any excess suicidality associated with specific antidepressants in adult populations. In fact, analysis of suicide items on depression rating scales show marked improvement in suicidal ideas with antidepressant treatment. Pharmacoepidemiology studies also have shown decreasing suicide rates associated with increasing rates of antidepressant prescriptions. However, overdose with venlafaxine has been shown to have greater propensity for deaths compared to SSRIs, but not as great as with TCAs.

In summary, unlike the youth age group (see Chapter 9), in adults there is no evidence that antidepressants cause an increase in suicidality overall. However, it is certainly possible that antidepressants can worsen suicidal ideation in a small subset of patients, perhaps by worsening anxiety and agitation. Therefore, it is important to carefully monitor clinical status, including suicidality, when initiating treatment. This is a period of high risk because patients are at high symptom severity, may not yet be feeling better from treatment, and instead may be experiencing troublesome side effects that contribute to suicidality.

6.4 **Drugs, doses, and common side effects**

43

6.4.1 **Selective serotonin reuptake inhibitors (SSRIs)**

The SSRIs are the most commonly prescribed antidepressants due to their tolerability, safety, simplicity of use, and broad spectrum efficacy. Although they share a common mechanism of action, the drugs in this class are not interchangeable for clinical efficacy or for side effect profile. This may be due to the different secondary receptor binding properties among these drugs. Fluoxetine and its active metabolite, norfluoxetine, have long half-lives (about 7 days, compared to 24 h for other SSRIs). Sertraline is associated with higher rates of diarrhea than other SSRIs. The SSRIs are generally weight neutral in acute trials, but paroxetine has greater weight gain with long-term use. Sexual side effects can occur in up to 40% of patients, especially ejaculation delay in men and orgasm delay in women, with more noticeable effects occurring with fluoxetine and paroxetine (Table 6.1).

Table 6.1 Selective serotonin reuptake inhibitors (SSRIs)

Mechanism of action	Common side effects (bold indicates >30%)	Drugs, usual daily doses	Comments
• Selective inhibition of serotonin reuptake	• GI (distress, nausea, vomiting, diarrhea)	• Citalopram, 20–60 mg	• Mild side effect profile, low potential for drug interactions
	• CNS (headache, agitation, sleep disturbance, tremor)	• Fluoxetine, 20–80 mg	• Longer half-life, markedly inhibits CYP 2D6, fewer discontinuation symptoms
	• Drowsiness, sedation, dry mouth	• Fluvoxamine, 100–300 mg	• More GI effects (**GI distress,** nausea) and sedation, markedly inhibits CYP 1A9
	• **Sexual side effects**	• Paroxetine, 20–60 mg	• More weight gain with long-term use, markedly inhibits CYP 2D6, more discontinuation symptoms (less so with CR formulation)
		• Sertraline, 50–200 mg	• More **diarrhea,** low potential for drug interactions

Abbreviations: CNS, central nervous system; CYP, Cytochrome P450; GI, gastrointestinal;

Table 6.2 Allosteric serotonin reuptake inhibitors (ASRIs)			
Mechanism of action	Common side effects (bold indicates >30%)	Drugs, usual daily doses	Comments
• Inhibition of serotonin reuptake • Allosteric binding to transporter protein	• Same as for SSRIs	• Escitalopram, 10–20 mg	• More effective than SSRIs, especially for more severely ill; mild side effects; low potential for drug interactions

6.4.2 **Allosteric serotonin reuptake inhibitors (ASRIs)**

The only medication in this class is escitalopram, the S-enantiomer of citalopram. Although it binds to the primary binding site on the serotonin transporter protein like the SSRIs, escitalopram is unique in that it also binds to an allosteric site on the transporter protein. The result of this allosteric binding is a more efficient inhibition of serotonin reuptake that increases serotonin availability in the synapse. This additional mechanism may explain the superior therapeutic effect of escitalopram over citalopram and other SSRIs. The side effect profile, however, is no different from that of citalopram (Table 6.2).

6.4.3 **Serotonin and noradrenaline reuptake inhibitors (SNRIs)**

Duloxetine and venlafaxine are examples of this class, which selectively inhibits serotonin and noradrenaline reuptake. Venlafaxine has a dose-dependent effect, with greater efficacy than SSRIs demonstrated when higher doses are used, perhaps because noradrenaline reuptake occurs only with doses greater than 150 mg/day. However, compared to SSRIs, venlafaxine has more side effects and discontinuations because of side effects, especially at higher doses. Venlafaxine is also associated with greater toxicity in overdose than other second-generation antidepressants, due to more cardiovascular effects (although this is not seen with therapeutic doses). Duloxetine has not shown the same superiority to SSRIs, but it has shown efficacy for diabetic neuropathic pain and also alleviates pain complaints associated with depression (Table 6.3).

6.4.4 **Other receptor agents**

These medications include mirtazapine and mianserin, which antagonize β_2 adrenergic autoreceptors, leading to increased release of serotonin and noradrenaline, and also block 5-HT$_{2C}$ receptors, which explains the lack of sexual and sleep side effects. Mirtazapine is also a potent histamine-1 receptor antagonist, which can help insomnia but also can result in anticholinergic side effects. Mirtazapine has more sedation, increased appetite, and weight gain compared to other second-generation antidepressants.

Table 6.3 Serotonin and noradrenaline reuptake inhibitors (SNRIs)

Mechanism of action	Common side effects (bold indicates >30%)	Drugs, usual daily doses	Comments
• Inhibition of serotonin reuptake • Inhibition of noradrenaline reuptake	• GI (distress, nausea, vomiting, diarrhea) • CNS (headache, agitation, sleep disturbance) • **Sexual side effects**	• Duloxetine, 60 mg • Venlafaxine-XR, 75–225 mg	• Less sexual dysfunction than SSRIs, effective in diabetic neuropathic pain • More effective than SSRIs • More **GI distress** and other side effects than SSRIs, dose-related increased blood pressure, less sexual dysfunction than SSRIs, more discontinuation symptoms (less so for XR formulation) • Less safe in overdose

Abbreviations: CNS, central nervous system; GI, gastrointestinal; SSRI, selective serotonin reuptake inhibitor

Bupropion is a noradrenaline and weak dopamine reuptake inhibitor. Because it has no effects on serotonin, its side effect profile is distinct from SSRIs, with fewer gastrointestinal (GI) and sexual side effects. It tends to be more activating, and unlike other antidepressants, does not show efficacy for anxiety disorders. Bupropion was associated with increased risk of seizures in patients with risk factors, but this has not been noted with the sustained and extended release formulations. Reboxetine is a selective noradrenaline reuptake inhibitor showing efficacy in depression. Atomoxetine is another selective noradrenaline reuptake inhibitor that is effective in attention deficit hyperactivity disorder, but there are no published studies in depression.

Agomelatine is a novel antidepressant that is an agonist of melatonin-1 and -2 receptors, and an antagonist of 5-HT_{2C} receptors. Besides efficacy in depressive symptoms, agomelatine shows greater beneficial effects on sleep architecture and symptoms than SSRIs and serotonin and noradrenaline reuptake inhibitors (SNRIs), with a side effect profile similar to that of placebo. Agomelatine also has fewer sexual side effects than SSRIs. The melatoninergic effects of agomelatine may also help regulate the sleep–wake cycle and other circadian rhythms (Table 6.4).

6.4.5 Tricyclic antidepressants (TCAs)

These drugs are still widely used but they have many limiting side effects and can be cardiotoxic even in therapeutic doses, and so are now usually considered second- or third-line choices. The tertiary amine TCAs (amitriptyline, imipramine) have more side effects because they also have active metabolites (nortriptyline and desipramine, respectively). One advantage for TCAs is that plasma drug concentrations have been correlated to therapeutic response and thus can be used to aid dose titration. Most have a minimum plasma concentration to achieve clinical response, but nortriptyline demonstrates a "therapeutic window" in that plasma levels above and below the therapeutic range are associated with lower response. Plasma drug concentration should not be used as a clinical indicator in overdose because of poor correlation with cardiotoxicity; electrocardiogram monitoring of QRS duration is a better predictor although it has, at best, moderate sensitivity and specificity (Table 6.5).

6.4.6 Monoamine oxidase inhibitors and related agents (MAOIs)

These drugs inhibit monoamine oxidase (MAO) A and B, which contributes to the metabolism of serotonin, noradrenaline, and dopamine. MAOIs are considered by many clinicians to be superior drugs for treatment-resistant depression, but the required dietary restrictions and potentially fatal drug interactions make them more difficult to use in clinical practice. Without MAO, tyramine found in

Table 6.4 Other receptor agents

Mechanism of action	Common side effects (bold indicates >30%)	Drugs, usual daily doses	Comments
• α₂-adrenergic autoreceptor antagonism • 5-HT₂c antagonism	• Fatigue, **drowsiness,** blurred vision, constipation, **weight gain**	• Mirtazapine, 15–45 mg • Mianserin, 30–90 mg	• Affects both serotonin and noradrenaline, beneficial effects on sleep, less sexual side effects than SSRIs • Antihistaminic properties result in increased appetite and **weight gain,** daytime sedation
• Inhibition of noradrenaline reuptake • Possible weak inhibition of dopamine reuptake	• Insomnia, agitation, dry mouth, blurred vision, constipation, sweating, tremor, GI distress	• Bupropion-SR, -XL, 300–400 mg	• Slight increased risk for seizures at higher doses, low rate of sexual side effects • Moderately inhibits CYP 2D6
• Selective inhibition of noradrenaline reuptake	• Dry mouth, constipation, insomnia, dizziness, tremor, sweating, urinary hesitancy, tachycardia	• Reboxetine, 4–10 mg	• At higher doses, urinary retention may occur
• Melatonin 1- and 2-receptor agonism • 5-HT₂c antagonism	• Dizziness, nausea, headache • Profile similar to placebo	• Agomelatine, 25–50 mg	• Beneficial effects on sleep, mild side effect profile, low rate of sexual side effects • May have beneficial chronobiotic properties

Abbreviations: CYP, cytochrome P450; GI, gastrointestinal; SSRI, selective serotonin reuptake inhibitor

Table 6.5 Tricyclic antidepressants (TCAs)

Mechanism of action	Common side effects (bold indicates >30%)	Drugs, usual daily doses	Comments
• Inhibition of serotonin reuptake • Inhibition of noradrenaline reuptake • Affects many other receptors (e.g., histamine, acetylcholine, β_2-adrenergic, etc)	• Side effects vary with drug—secondary amine TCAs have fewer side effects than tertiary amine • Anticholinergic (blurred vision, **dry mouth**, constipation, urinary retention, sweating, confusion) • Antihistaminic (**drowsiness, sedation**, weight gain) • Cardiovascular (dizziness, postural hypotension, antiarrhythmic effects, QRS prolongation) • GI (nausea, vomiting) • CNS (tremor, headaches, seizures, insomnia) • **Sexual dysfunction**	*Secondary amines* • Nortriptyline, 75–150 mg • Desipramine, 75–225 mg • Dothiepin, 75–300 mg *Tertiary amines* • Amitriptyline, 75–300 mg • Imipramine, 100–300 mg • Clomipramine, 100–300 mg *Heterocyclic* • Maprotiline, 100–225 mg • Amoxapine, 200–400 mg • Lofepramine, 140–210 mg	• Fewest anticholinergic/CV effects • Therapeutic window for plasma level • More activating • Minimum therapeutic plasma level • Similar to desipramine • Most sedating, used in low doses as hypnotic, used for pain • Minimum therapeutic plasma level • Very sedating • Minimum therapeutic plasma level • More effective in severe depression, used for OCD, very sedating • Minimum therapeutic plasma level • Lowers seizure threshold • Dopaminergic, may be useful in psychotic depression, but also more likely to cause EPS • Although it is metabolized to desipramine, it has a safe CV profile, even in overdose

Abbreviations: CV, cardiovascular; EPS, extrapyramidal syndromes; GI, gastrointestinal

CHAPTER 6 **Pharmacotherapy**

certain foods (ripe cheese, red wine) is not metabolized, and can result in hypertensive crises. Serotonergic syndrome has also occurred from combining MAOIs with serotonergic antidepressants and other agents. Because they irreversibly inhibit MAO, a 2-week washout is necessary when switching from an MAOI to another antidepressant to allow for regeneration of MAO. Similarly, a 1-week washout (5 weeks for fluoxetine) is required when switching from another antidepressant to an MAOI.

Moclobemide, a reversible inhibitor of MAO-A, does not require the same dietary restrictions because MAO-B is still available for metabolizing tyramine. Moclobemide has a benign side effect profile but many clinicians do not regard it as potent as MAOIs.

Selegiline (also known as deprenyl) is a selective, irreversible MAO-B inhibitor that is available as a transdermal delivery system (patch). At lower doses it does not require dietary restrictions, but at higher doses (and with overdose) selegiline loses selectivity and acts as an MAOI, thereby requiring a tyramine-free diet. Both selegiline and moclobemide carry the same cautions for drug interactions as for the MAOIs (Table 6.6).

6.5 Drug interactions

Some antidepressants can inhibit a specific cytochrome P450 (CYP) isoenzyme, thereby leading to increased blood levels of concurrent drugs that are metabolized by that isoenzyme (Table 6.7). For example, fluoxetine and paroxetine markedly inhibit CYP 2D6, which extensively metabolizes several TCAs. If these TCAs are concurrently taken with fluoxetine or paroxetine, plasma TCA levels can increase by as much as 5–10 times than usual for a given dose. Thus, a 200 mg dose essentially becomes equivalent to a 2,000 mg dose, which can be cardiotoxic. Therefore, lower TCA doses must be prescribed and plasma TCA levels carefully monitored when used concurrently with fluoxetine or paroxetine.

6.6 Switching

Many patients will need to be switched from one antidepressant to another for nonresponse or intolerance. Switching involves consideration of potential side effects, discontinuation effects, drug interactions, and rapidity of switch. It is usually not necessary to stop the first antidepressant before starting the second (the V approach, see Figure 6.1). Instead, the first antidepressant can be tapered down while the second is tapered up (the X approach). The advantage of the X approach is that it takes much less time. The disadvantages include the possibility of additive side effects and difficulty differentiating discontinuation symptoms (from the first drug) from side effects of the second drug.

Table 6.6 Monoamine oxidase inhibitors (MAOIs) and related agents

Mechanism of action	Common side effects (bold indicates >30%)	Drugs, usual daily doses	Comments
• Irreversible inhibition of MAO (A and B)	• **Hypertensive crises** • Drowsiness, agitation, hyper-reflexia, headache, sweating, GI distress, weight gain, sleep disturbance, orthostatic hypotension, edema	• Phenelzine, 45–90 mg • Tranylcypromine, 30–60 mg	• Phenelzine more sedating, tranylcypromine more activating • MAOIs require tyramine-free diet • Caution for drug interactions (see Table 6.7) • Requires 2-week washout before switching to another drug
		• Isocarboxazid, 20–60 mg	• Milder side effects compared to other MAOIs
• Reversible inhibition of MAO-A	• Insomnia, agitation, headache, sedation, dry mouth, constipation, nausea, dizziness	• Moclobemide, 300–600 mg	• Mild side effect profile, dietary restrictions not needed • Same cautions for drug interactions as for MAOIs
• Selective irreversible inhibition of MAO-B	• Application site reactions, insomnia, headache, dry mouth, diarrhea	• Selegiline transdermal patch, 6–12 mg	• At higher doses and in overdosage, selegiline also inhibits MAO-A, thereby acting as an MAOI • Dietary restrictions not needed for 6 mg dose, but tyramine-free diet recommended for 9–12 mg dose • Same cautions for drug interactions as for MAOIs

Abbreviations: GI, gastrointestinal; MAO, monoamine oxidase

Table 6.7 Clinically significant interactions of antidepressants with common drugs*

Drug	Mechanism	Interacts with	Comments
Fluoxetine	• Marked inhibition of CYP 2D6	• TCAs • Beta blockers (metoprolol, propranolol) • Codeine and other opioids (reduces effect)	• Can potentially increase serum TCA levels to cardiotoxic levels • Long half-life of fluoxetine means that inhibition of CYP 2D6 can occur for up to 5 weeks after discontinuation
Paroxetine	• Marked inhibition of CYP 2D6	• TCAs • Beta blockers (metoprolol, propranolol) • Codeine and other opioids (reduces effect)	• Can potentially increase serum TCA levels to cardiotoxic levels
Bupropion	• Moderate inhibition of CYP 2D6	• TCAs • Beta blockers (metoprolol, propranolol) • Codeine and other opioids (reduces effect)	• Usually not a clinically relevant effect, but caution with higher doses
Duloxetine	• Moderate inhibition of CYP 2D6	• TCAs • Beta blockers (metoprolol, propranolol) • Codeine and other opioids (reduces effect)	• Usually not a clinically relevant effect, but caution with higher doses
Fluvoxamine	• Marked inhibition of CYP 1A2 • Moderate inhibition of CYP 3A4 • Moderate inhibition of CYP 2C19	• Buspirone • Clozapine • Diazepam • Quinidine • Warfarin • Statin drugs • Sildenafil • Vardenafil • Phenytoin • Cyclosporine	• Increased statin levels can cause rhabdomyolysis • Monitor INR carefully when warfarin used

Table 6.7 (Contd.)			
MAOIs (isocar- boxazid, phenelzine, tranyl- cypromine)	• Inhibits MAO metabolism of noradrenaline, serotonin and dopamine	• High tyramine-containing foods • Sympathomi- metic agents (e.g., pseudo- ephedrine) • Meperidine • Dextro- morphan • Other antidepressants • Other serotonergic agents	• Potentially fatal reactions with sympathomimet- ics or tyramine due to hyper- tensive crises • Delirium, confu- sion, seizures, coma, death reported after ingestion of meperidine or other narcotics (including dex- tromorphan), and with sero- tonergic agents • Avoid disulfiram (Antabuse) with isocarboxazid
Moclo- bemide	• Inhibits MAO metabolism of noradrenaline, serotonin and dopamine	• Same as for MAOIs (except dietary interactions)	• Theoretical risk of serotonin syndrome
Selegiline	• Inhibits MAO metabolism of noradrenaline, serotonin and dopamine	• Same as for MAOIs (except dietary interac- tions at lower doses)	• Theoretical risk of serotonin syndrome
TCAs	• Substrate for CYP 2D6	• Fluoxetine • Paroxetine • Bupropion (less likely)	• Can potentially increase serum TCA levels to cardiotoxic levels

*Not a comprehensive list of interactions, only a selection of commonly used drugs.
Marked: >150% increase in blood levels; moderate: 50–150% increase in blood levels.
Abbreviations: CYP, cytochrome P450; MAO, monoamine oxidase; MAOI, monoamine oxidase inhibitor; TCA, tricyclic antidepressant

53

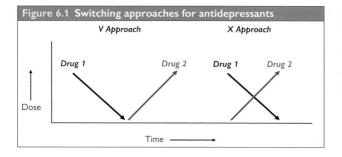

Figure 6.1 Switching approaches for antidepressants

V Approach   X Approach

Drug 1   Drug 2   Drug 1   Drug 2

Dose

Time ⟶

Washout periods are usually not required for switching between most antidepressants, especially the SSRIs and newer medications (Table 6.8). The exception is switching to or from MAOIs. When switching to an MAOI, the first drug should be washed out (at least 1 week for most antidepressants, 5 weeks for fluoxetine). When switching from an MAOI to another antidepressant, a 2-week washout is necessary to ensure that endogenous MAO is regenerated. For the reversible inhibitor of monoamine oxidase-A (RIMA), moclobemide, and the selective MAO–B inhibitor, selegiline, only 1 week is necessary for washout when switching to another antidepressant.

Table 6.8 Washout periods required for switching between antidepressants

Switching to:	SSRIs/ASRI	SNRIs and other agents	TCAs	MAOIs	Moclobemide selegiline
Switching from:					
SSRIs/ ASRI	None (watch for additive serotonergic effects)	None (watch for additive serotonergic effects)	None (watch for additive serotonergic effects)	1 week (5 weeks for fluoxetine)	1 week (5 weeks for fluoxetine
SNRIs and other newer agents	None (watch for additive serotonergic effects)	None (watch for additive serotonergic/ noradrenergic effects)	None (watch for additive serotonergic/ noradrenergic effects)	1 week	1 week
TCAs	None (watch for additive serotonergic effects)	None (watch for additive serotonergic/ noradrenergic effects)	None (watch for additive serotonergic/ noradrenergic effects)	1 week	1 week
MAOIs	2 weeks	2 weeks	2 weeks	2 weeks	2 weeks
Moclobemide/ selegiline	1 week	1 week	1 week	1 week	1 week

Abbreviations: ASRI, allosteric serotonin reuptake inhibitor; MAOI, monoamine oxidase inhibitor; SNRI, serotonin and noradrenaline reuptake inhibitor; SSRI, selective serotonin reuptake inhibitor; TCA, tricyclic antidepressant

Box 6.1 **FINISH mnemonic* for antidepressant discontinuation symptoms**	
F	Flu-like symptoms
I	Insomnia
N	Nausea
I	Imbalance
S	Sensory disturbances
H	Hyperarousal (agitation)

*Adapted from Berber MJ. *J Clin Psychiatry* 1998; **59**:255.

6.7 **Discontinuation**

Some patients will experience discontinuation symptoms (Box 6.1), usually of mild severity, when antidepressants are abruptly stopped. Paroxetine, venlafaxine, and TCAs are most likely to be associated with discontinuation symptoms (but less so with the controlled and extended release preparations), while fluoxetine is the least likely, in part due to its long half-life. Other drugs with low propensity for discontinuation symptoms include agomelatine, bupropion, citalopram, escitalopram, moclobemide, and sertraline.

While discontinuation symptoms are not true withdrawal syndromes and the symptoms are usually transient, they may be quite uncomfortable. Whenever possible, tapering medications slowly (by one dose level every week) is prudent. If necessary, reinstating the dose will ameliorate the symptoms. For those patients who have difficulty stopping the drug even when on the minimum dose, tapering to alternate day dosing may be helpful.

Key references

Bezchlibnyk-Butler KZ, Jeffries JJ. *Clinical Handbook of Psychotropic Drugs*, 16th revised edition. Toronto: Hogrefe and Huber, 2006.

CINP Task Force. *The Use and Usefulness of Antidepressants: A Technical Review of Evidence by a Task Force Report of the CINP*. Geneva: Collegium Internationale Neuro-psychopharmacologicum, 2006.

Ebmeier KP, Donaghey C, Steele JD. Recent developments and current controversies in depression. *Lancet* 2006; **367**:153–67.

Gartlehner G, Hansen RA, Thieda P, *et al.* Comparative effectiveness of second-generation antidepressants in the pharmacologic treatment of adult depression. *Comparative Effectiveness Review No.7*. Rockville MD: Agency for Healthcare Research and Quality, 2007.

Kennedy SH, Lam RW, Cohen NL, Ravindran AV, CANMAT Depression Work Group. Clinical guidelines for the treatment of depressive disorders. IV. Medications and other biological treatments. *Can J Psychiatry* 2001; **46**(Suppl 1):38S–58S.

Simon GE. How can we know whether antidepressants increase suicide risk? *Am J Psychiatry* 2006; **163**: 1861–3.

Stahl SM. *Essential Psychopharmacology of Depression and Bipolar Disorder.* Cambridge: Cambridge University Press, 2001.

Vasa RA, Carlino AR, Pine DS. Pharmacotherapy of depressed children and adolescents: current issues and potential directions. *Biol Psychiatry* 2006; **59**:1021–8.

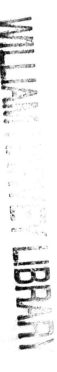

Chapter 7

Somatic treatments

> **Key points**
> - Wake therapy, exercise, and light therapy are non-invasive and clinically useful treatments.
> - Electroconvulsive therapy remains an effective, safe, and well-tolerated treatment for patients with severe, psychotic, or medication-resistant depression.
> - Repetitive transcranial magnetic stimulation is an emerging treatment with increasing evidence for acute efficacy, but with limited data about long-term management.
> - Surgical treatments with novel neuromodulation techniques may become clinically useful for some patients with difficult-to-treat depression.

7.1 Introduction

Psychiatry has a long history of using physical or somatic treatments that purport to address the biological pathogenesis of depression. One of the earliest and best-known of these somatic treatments is electroconvulsive therapy (ECT), which, despite the negative popularized depictions of its use, remains one of the safest and most effective treatments for severe and treatment-resistant depression (TRD, see Chapter 9). Others, such as insulin shock, are no longer used because the risks of treatment outweighed any proven benefits. Somatic treatments, however, vary from non-invasive (wake therapy, exercise, light therapy) to more invasive methods (transcranial magnetic stimulation) and to the most invasive (those that involve surgery such as vagus nerve stimulation (VNS), limbic neurosurgery).

A major problem for evaluating somatic treatments is that, since a physical treatment is used, designing a suitable placebo control condition for randomized controlled trials (RCTs) is challenging, and blinding of conditions is often very difficult to achieve. Hence, the evidence base for these somatic treatments is not as robust as for medication treatments (Table 7.1).

Table 7.1 Level of evidence supporting efficacy of somatic treatments

Somatic treatment	Level of evidence*
Wake therapy (sleep deprivation)	• RCTs (not sham-controlled)
Exercise	• Small-sample RCTs (sham-controlled)
Light therapy	• RCTs (sham-controlled) • Meta-analyses
Repetitive transcranial magnetic stimulation	• RCTs (sham-controlled) • Meta-analyses
Electroconvulsive therapy	• RCTs (sham-controlled) • Meta-analyses
Vagus nerve stimulation	• Large prospective cohort studies
Deep brain stimulation	• Small-sample case series
Limbic neurosurgery	• Prospective case series

* RCTs: randomized controlled trials.

7.2 **Wake therapy (sleep deprivation)**

As disturbances in the sleep–wake cycle are cardinal symptoms of major depressive disorder (MDD), it is not surprising that manipulation of the sleep–wake cycle has been investigated as a treatment. What may be surprising, however, is that although depressed patients complain of insomnia and resulting daytime fatigue, keeping them awake all night can result in a clear improvement in mood that continues through the next day. Total sleep deprivation (TSD, now known as wake therapy to better describe the active intervention) can result in dramatic changes in mood, with many patients feeling a return to baseline. Although it is difficult to design placebo-controlled studies, the fact that wake therapy is so counterintuitive to patients (most of whom think they will feel better if only they had *more* sleep) makes a placebo response less likely.

Unfortunately, the mood improvement after TSD is not long-lived. The majority of patients relapse after a recovery sleep the next day after TSD. Several reviews of sleep deprivation studies found the clinical response rate to TSD averaged about 60%, but 80–85% of patients relapsed the next day after the recovery sleep. Relapse can occur even after brief naps. However, it is intriguing that up to 15% of patients appear to have sustained responses to TSD even after a recovery sleep. Newer techniques have suggested that wake therapy, in combination with medications such as lithium or antidepressants, or with bright light therapy, can help sustain response in a good proportion of patients. The main problem with wake therapy is adherence, as many patients do not have the motivation to stay awake all night. A regimen in which an all night sleep deprivation is alternated with nights of regular sleep may make it easier to perform as an outpatient. Alternatively, partial sleep deprivation, in which patients are allowed to sleep from 10 pm to 2 am, may also be effective and may make it easier for patients to comply with wake therapy.

Clinical summary: Given the non-invasive, easily conducted nature of wake therapy, it can be considered as adjunctive treatment for patients with MDD, especially those who require rapid response and can be monitored (e.g., hospitalized patients, acutely suicidal patients).

7.3 Exercise

Exercise has been shown to improve mood and reduce depressive symptoms, with some (methodologically limited) studies suggesting an antidepressant effect of the same magnitude as cognitive therapy. More recent studies have shown that young and elderly individuals who engage in programs of exercise display fewer depressive symptoms and are less likely to subsequently develop MDD. Three recent studies in MDD found that exercise significantly improved depression, as monotherapy and as adjunctive to medication, and that moderate aerobic exercise was more effective than low-intensity exercise or flexibility exercise.

Clinical summary: Although the evidence for exercise as monotherapy for MDD is limited, it seems reasonable to recommend regular exercise as adjunctive treatment.

7.4 Light therapy

Light therapy consists of daily exposure to bright, artificial light, usually administered with a fluorescent light box. Light therapy has been found to be effective in seasonal affective disorder (in DSM-IV TR terminology: recurrent major depressive episodes with a seasonal pattern) and has been studied in other conditions such as nonseasonal depression, bulimia nervosa, and premenstrual depressive disorder.

The standard protocol for light therapy is 10,000 lux white, fluorescent light (with ultraviolet wavelengths blocked) for 30 min a day in the early morning upon arising from sleep. Newer light treatment devices include those using light-emitting diodes (LEDs). These have the advantage of long life, portability due to less power needs and can be battery-powered, and differences in wavelength that may be

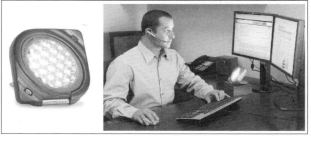

Figure 7.1 Example of an LED device and its use for light therapy

more efficient (Figure 7.1). Light therapy devices (costing about US$120–300) are available for purchase at local medical equipment stores or on the Internet.

The effect of light therapy is mediated through the eyes to the brain via the retinohypothalamic tract. Major hypotheses for its therapeutic effect involve circadian rhythm regulation (light is the strongest synchronizer of the circadian pacemaker in the brain, located in the suprachiasmatic nucleus of the hypothalamus) or effects on neurotransmitter dysregulation (particularly serotonin or dopamine). Several systematic reviews of RCTs, including one for the Cochrane Collaboration, have shown that bright light is effective in the treatment of seasonal depression, with some trials showing the effects of light to be comparable to selective serotonin reuptake inhibitor (SSRI) antidepressants. However, there is still only limited evidence for the efficacy of light therapy in other conditions, including nonseasonal depression.

Adverse effects reported for light therapy are generally mild, but include headache, nausea, eyestrain, agitation, and insomnia. There are also case reports of manic induction with bright light so that patients with bipolar disorder should use the same cautions as with other antidepressants. Relative contraindications to using bright light include pre-existing retinal disease, macular degeneration, and use of retinal photosensitizing drugs (e.g., thioridazine, lithium, melatonin).

Clinical summary: Light therapy is a first-line treatment for seasonal affective disorder. Although the evidence base for efficacy in nonseasonal depression is limited, given the non-invasive nature, tolerability, and low cost of light therapy, it can be considered as a first-line treatment for patients with mild to moderate depression severity when standard treatments are not tolerated, or as adjunctive treatment with antidepressants.

7.5 **Transcranial magnetic stimulation**

Repetitive transcranial magnetic stimulation (rTMS) is a technique in which a brief, high intensity magnetic field is generated and used to stimulate cortical neurons. The advantage of rTMS is that it is a non-invasive treatment that can be applied while patients are awake, and in which adverse effects are minimal. Compared to ECT, there are no cognitive side effects and no anesthesia is required. In the mid-1990s, rTMS, in which a "train" of sequential pulses is applied in one session, began to be evaluated as a treatment for neuropsychiatric conditions. Since then, dozens of studies and several systematic reviews have found statistically significant effects of active rTMS over sham control conditions. However, the clinical relevance of these findings is not as clear, as the overall clinical response of rTMS (whether measured as percentage improvement on depression rating scales or as dichotomous outcomes on global improvement scales) has been rather limited. In part, this may have been due to inclusion of early studies in which stimulus parameters were still being investigated and optimized.

More recently, there has been consensus that high frequency stimulation over the left dorsolateral prefrontal cortex (DLPFC) or low frequency stimulation over the right DLPFC are associated with antidepressant effects. Consequently, recent trials with these stimulus parameters have shown greater clinical effect than previous studies. Several studies in TRD have also shown benefit of rTMS over sham conditions. Direct comparisons with ECT have shown similar efficacy, although these were not placebo controlled.

The major limitation for evidence of rTMS in efficacy is longer term follow-up. The studies of rTMS have been short—1 to 4 weeks in duration—and it is unclear how long the therapeutic effects last. In fact, one systematic review for the Cochrane Collaboration found no difference between active and sham conditions at 2 weeks following treatment. Thus, it is unclear how rTMS fits into the management of depression.

Clinical summary: rTMS is an emerging treatment with few side effects and efficacy demonstrated in very short term studies, but data on longer term outcomes are not available and it remains unclear how to manage responders to treatment. Further studies are required before rTMS can be recommended for general clinical use.

7.6 **Electroconvulsive therapy**

ECT remains one of the most effective treatments in psychiatry, with response rates of 60–90%, and recent developments in ECT have optimized the treatment parameters while reducing cognitive side effects. ECT also appears to work faster than antidepressants, especially for elderly patients and those with psychotic depression. Systematic reviews have highlighted the strong evidence for efficacy compared to sham treatments and recent RCTs have also shown clear acute benefits of ECT. Unfortunately, there are still few comparisons of ECT with second-generation antidepressants and combinations.

Indications for ECT are shown in Box 7.1. High-dose (three to eight times the dose needed for seizure threshold) unilateral electrode placement has similar efficacy to bilateral placement with fewer cognitive side effects. There is also some evidence that bifrontal electrode placement, which requires lower electrical dose to achieve seizures, also has similar efficacy to the traditional bitemporal placement, with fewer cognitive side effects. Seizure duration is commonly monitored using EEG or the blood pressure cuff method (for seizure-induced motor activity) but there is no good definition of an "adequate" seizure. The usual course of treatment consists of 6–12 sessions administered three times a week, but less frequent sessions are associated with fewer cognitive side effects.

ECT is a safe treatment. With careful pre-anesthesia examination, the mortality rate approximates that of general anesthesia. There is no evidence for any long-term neural damage due to ECT, and in fact there are animal studies suggesting that electroconvulsive shock can lead to enhanced neurogenesis. Combining antidepressants with ECT is not more effective than ECT alone during acute treatment. As an ineffective pre-ECT medication will not be useful for maintenance and may contribute to additive side effects, antidepressants should be discontinued before or during a course of ECT, and starting a new agent should wait till the completion of the ECT course.

The common side effects of ECT relate to recovery from the general anesthetic and the brief seizure, including nausea, headache, and muscle aches. These resolve spontaneously or with symptomatic treatment. Less common are musculoskeletal and dental injuries,

> ### Box 7.1 Indications for electroconvulsive therapy (ECT) in depression
>
> - High suicide potential
> - Deteriorating physical status (e.g., inability to eat or drink)
> - Psychotic features (especially delusional depression)
> - Previous good response to ECT
> - Poor response to antidepressants
> - Inability to tolerate antidepressants
> - Pregnancy
> - Patient preference

persistent myalgia, and cardiovascular events. The cognitive side effects of ECT include a post-ECT confusional state (due to post-ictal and post-anesthetic effects) that resolves quickly, and a short-term retrograde memory loss that resolves more slowly. Although there are anecdotal reports of severe and permanent memory loss, neuro-psychological studies show no sustained cognitive deficits with testing 6 months following ECT. Some loss of memory for events surround-ing the time of ECT may linger, but longer term cognitive effects seem to be selective for impersonal autobiographical memories (such as public events) that do not affect function. In addition, the majority of patients show improvement in cognitive function because their depression-related memory problems improve.

Without maintenance treatment, relapse following successful ECT is high, ranging from 50–80% within 6 months. Greater severity and degree of medication-resistance is associated with higher rate of relapse. There are limited data on maintenance options, but the combination of lithium and nortriptyline was found to be superior to nortriptyline alone, and continuation ECT (starting at twice a month and then tapering to once a month) was also as effective as the lith-ium-nortriptyline combination.

Clinical summary: ECT is a safe and effective treatment that should be considered in the treatment algorithm for TRD, psychotic depression, and severely compromised patients. The transient memory disturbance associated with ECT can be minimized using high-dose unilateral or lower-dose bifrontal electrode placement. Maintenance strategies, including antidepressants, combination of lithium-nortriptyline and continuation ECT, are important to prevent relapse following ECT.

7.7 Surgical treatments

7.7.1 Vagus nerve stimulation

VNS involves surgical implantation of an electrode around the left vagus nerve in the neck, connected to a stimulator/battery pack, similar to a pacemaker, implanted under the chest wall. Electrical stimulation to the vagus nerve is continuously applied in a cycle of 30 s on, 5 min off. A major advantage of VNS is that compliance to treatment is 100%.

VNS is an effective and approved treatment for medication-refractory epilepsy, but when study patients were found to have improved mood independent of effects on seizures, VNS was investi-gated for TRD. Initial open-label pilot studies were encouraging, but an 8-week double-blind RCT did not find any effects of active VNS compared to inactive. However, patients with activated VNS contin-ued to improve over a 1–2 year naturalistic follow-up, and outcomes were better than a matched cohort of patients with TRD that

Chapter 8

Psychotherapy

> **Key points**
> - Evidenced-based psychotherapies for depression include problem-solving therapy, cognitive behaviour therapy, interpersonal psychotherapy, and cognitive behavioural-analysis system of psychotherapy.
> - For mild to moderate severity of depression, evidence-based psychotherapies are first-line treatments and are as effective as pharmacotherapy.
> - For more severe, chronic or comorbid depressions, combined treatment with psychotherapy and pharmacotherapy is indicated.
> - Cognitive therapy may provide additional and enduring benefits to prevent relapse or recurrence.

8.1 Introduction

8.11 Efficacy

Evidenced-based psychotherapies are those that have shown empirical evidence of efficacy in randomized controlled trials (RCTs) in defined populations of patients with major depressive disorder (MDD). Table 8.1 lists the evidence-based psychotherapies and their key features. Although these psychotherapies have different principles, areas of focus, and techniques, they also share many common elements, including their short-term nature, active participation by both therapist and patient, and use of pragmatic strategies. Other psychotherapies (e.g., psychodynamic psychotherapy) may also be effective for MDD but have not been systematically studied, and so are considered second- or third-line recommendations.

Many therapists in the community use an assortment of techniques from different types of psychotherapy in what is sometimes termed "eclectic psychotherapy." However, some evidence suggests that the more experienced the therapist, and the greater the integrity of the therapist to the structure of a particular psychotherapy, the better is the outcome. Access to evidence-based psychotherapies is still a major problem for patients, as the availability of qualified therapists is limited, and psychotherapy is often not funded by public health systems.

Table 8.1 Key features of evidence-based psychotherapies for depression

Psychotherapy	Main principles	Duration	Comments
Problem-solving therapy (PST)	• Identify problems • Develop problem solving skills	4–6 sessions	Developed for primary care settings
Cognitive Therapy (CT)	• Identify patterns of negative thinking and attitudes • Challenge faulty beliefs • Substitute more rational thoughts	12–16 sessions	Often used with BT as Cognitive-behaviour therapy (CBT).
Behaviour Therapy (BT)	• Identify maladaptive patterns of behaviour • Reinforce positive coping behaviours • Use social skills training	8–12 sessions	Often used with CT as Cognitive-behaviour therapy (CBT).
Interpersonal Psychotherapy (IPT)	• Identify major interpersonal issues • Use practical strategies to deal with one or two issues	12–16 sessions	Uses cognitive/behavioural and psychodynamic techniques.
Cognitive Behavioural-Analysis System of Psychotherapy (CBASP)	• Analyze specific situations which led to interpersonal problems • Use problem solving techniques to develop alternate ways of dealing with interpersonal situations	16–20 sessions	Developed specifically for chronic depression.

8.1.2 Choice of psychotherapy

There are very few comparison studies of evidence-based psychotherapies. Meta-analyses have shown that CBT and IPT have similar effect sizes and perform equally well in MDD. There is also little information about clinical factors that might predict better outcomes with a specific psychotherapy. In one of the few large trials comparing CT and IPT, the predictive factors found for response were counterintuitive—namely, that patients did better with CT when they had fewer negative cognitions while patients did better with IPT when they had less social impairment. Several studies have shown that investigator allegiance to a particular psychotherapy also influences outcomes.

8.1.3 Psychotherapy and pharmacotherapy

Most comparisons of psychotherapies with pharmacotherapy have been conducted in patients with MDD of mild to moderate severity. The overall conclusion from RCTs and meta-analyses is that evidence-based psychotherapies are as effective as antidepressants for these patients. There are few studies of psychotherapy for severe depression, but CT was found to be of similar efficacy to paroxetine (with or without augmentation using lithium and desipramine) in one recent trial (although pharmacotherapy showed numerically higher response and remission rates). Most clinicians would still recommend combined treatment with psychotherapy and pharmacotherapy for severe, comorbid, and chronic depression.

Non-response to either psychotherapy or to pharmacotherapy does not imply general refractoriness to treatment. That is, patients who have not responded to psychotherapy will show typical response rates to pharmacotherapy, and vice versa. It does not appear that psychotherapy and pharmacotherapy target the same mechanisms.

8.2 Problem-solving therapy

Problem-solving therapy (PST) is a brief treatment that was developed for use in primary care settings and is closely related to CBT. PST consists of 4–6 sessions of 20–30 min each that teach a structured approach to identifying problems and using pragmatic problem-solving techniques. These include breaking down problems into manageable components, sorting priorities, brainstorming solutions, and listing advantages and disadvantages for potential solutions. Several large, pragmatic RCTs have shown superior outcomes with PST compared to treatment as usual for MDD in primary care practices. One advantage of PST is it can be delivered by health care workers who do not specialize in mental health (such as nurses, family physicians, care managers, etc.) and only brief training is required. Therefore, PST could become more widely available than other therapies that need more extensive training and experience.

8.3 Cognitive-behavioural therapy

8.3.1 Cognitive therapy

Cognitive therapy (CT) is the most validated psychosocial treatment in psychiatry, with numerous RCTs and meta-analyses showing evidence for efficacy in MDD. In CT, automatic negative thoughts associated with depression are believed to underlie the depressive feelings and affect. These negative thoughts are formulated into dysfunctional attitudes about the self, others, and the world. CT seeks to systematically identify these thinking patterns (such as, I'm always a failure) and then rationally challenge them (e.g., How can you tell if you are a failure? What evidence is there that you are a failure? Is there any evidence that you are NOT a failure?). Table 8.2 illustrates other examples of negative cognitions.

Techniques of CT include keeping track of automatic thoughts, assessing the affect associated with them, and then reassessing feelings after an intervention such as a rational challenge. The therapist uses an active Socratic questioning style to teach the client how to substitute more rational thoughts. Homework assignment and review is an integral part of CT.

CT also appears to have enduring effects beyond acute treatment. In studies of treatment discontinuation, patients who stopped CT after acute treatment had lower relapse rates on long-term follow-up than those who were discontinued from medications. The relapse/recurrence rates following CT given only in the acute phase of treatment were similar to patients who continued on maintenance medications. Similarly, CT has been shown to reduce relapse/recurrence when given after an acute course of antidepressants, even if the medication is discontinued. Thus, it appears that CT reduces vulnerability to further depression while medications appear to provide only symptomatic relief. It is unclear whether this is due to compensatory mechanisms (e.g., learning new ways to adapt to depressive symptomatology) or whether there is a fundamental change in the processes that are causal for depression (e.g., changing negative cognitive schemas).

8.3.2 Behaviour therapy

Behaviour therapy (BT) is also a widely validated treatment for MDD. BT is based on the principle that depression is associated with a decrease in goal-directed behaviours and reduction of positive reinforcing activities. This sets up a "vicious circle" in which reduced activity leads to more inertia that further limits activity. In BT, the

Table 8.2 Examples of negative cognitions	
Minimizing/maximizing	I never have any fun anymore; winning the lottery just means more people will come after me for money
Catastrophizing	If I don't go to the office party, no one at work will speak to me again
Negative inference	My boss didn't give me a good assignment, which proves that he doesn't like me
Over-generalizing	I heard someone say that I am shy, so I can't make any friends
Dichotomous (black and white) thinking	If I don't get an A on this report, I'm not worthy of graduate school
Over-personalization	If my daughter loses the spelling contest, I must be a bad father

inertia and reduction in goal-directed activities are addressed to facilitate new learned behaviours. Negative behaviours (such as crying or angry tirades) are also targeted. Various activation techniques are used, including increasing the number of pleasurable activities, tracking moods, relaxation exercises and social skills training. The emphasis is on mastery of situations and skills. As in CT, monitoring mood and affect and doing homework are essential components of BT. In one RCT for severe depression, BT was found to be as effective as antidepressant medication, and both were superior to CT alone.

8.3.3 Cognitive-behaviour therapy

Cognitive therapy and behaviour therapy are often used together as cognitive-behaviour therapy (CBT), especially in community practice. CBT is also widely used in other psychiatric and medical conditions. A recent adaption of CBT, incorporating mindfulness-based meditation techniques, has shown promise in preventing relapse in patients with recurrent MDD.

Workbooks and patient guides to CBT have long been available, but a new development in CBT is the use of Internet and computer-assisted programs to deliver CBT. Preliminary studies suggest that these may be effective interventions for MDD, which would make CBT much more accessible to patients.

8.4 Interpersonal psychotherapy

Interpersonal psychotherapy (IPT) is based on the observation that people with depression, whether as a contributory cause or a consequence, often have disturbed interpersonal relationships. IPT was developed in conjunction with pharmacotherapy and uses an explicit medical model for illness. In IPT, the therapeutic focus is on four common interpersonal issues (Table 8.3). The initial stage of IPT begins with an extensive interpersonal history to identify which of these problems is relevant for the patient, and to decide on which one or two issues to work on. IPT is much less structured than CBT, but the focus on pragmatic methods means that many cognitive and behavioural techniques are used in IPT.

| Table 8.3 Issues and strategies in interpersonal psychotherapy ||
Interpersonal issue	Strategies
Unresolved grief	Encourage reminiscing, undergo mourning, consider future planning
Relationship conflict (e.g., marital problems)	Problem solve, learn communication and conflict resolution skills
Role transition (e.g., empty-nesters, divorce, loss of job, retirement)	Consider both losses and benefits of transition, use activation techniques
Social isolation	Learn and practice social skills

8.5 **Cognitive behavioural-analysis system of psychotherapy**

The cognitive behavioural-analysis system of psychotherapy (CBASP) was developed specifically for chronic depression and includes elements of both CBT and psychodynamic psychotherapy. CBASP is based on the assumption that patients with chronic depression are perceptually disconnected from their environmental situations so that consequences are not appropriately reinforcing behaviours. The first phase of CBASP is a detailed personal history of interpersonal relationships, often identifying traumatic events and stressful relationships. Using a technique termed situational analysis, the therapist helps the patient to identify the effects of their behaviours on others, and also uses the therapist–patient interaction to illustrate these effects. The therapy then uses behavioural skills training and rehearsal to modify the consequences of behaviours and change the interpersonal dynamic.

In a large ($N = 681$), 20-week RCT of patients with chronic MDD, CBASP was as effective as an antidepressant (nefazodone, unfortunately no longer available due to problems with liver toxicity), but the combination of antidepressant plus CBASP was significantly better than either monotherapy (75% remission rates compared to less than 50% for the monotherapies). Therefore, patients are encouraged to use pharmacotherapy as they undergo CBASP.

8.6 **Group psychotherapies**

Most of the individual psychotherapies can be adapted to couples or group settings, and both CBT and IPT are available in group formats. Marital therapy, which usually incorporates CBT or IPT techniques, also has been shown to be effective for MDD. The advantages of group psychotherapy are that participants have more sources for support and encouragement during stressful situations; a group offers the opportunity to practice interpersonal techniques and receive feedback, and groups may be more cost-effective. Some of the potential disadvantages of group psychotherapy are that often patients will prefer individual therapy (which may, in part, be a consequence of their depressive symptoms, i.e., social isolation and anxiety), individual therapy may be more effective, and it is more difficult to engage patients and schedule appointments for groups.

8.7 **Maintenance and prevention**

CT has been shown to have some enduring effects after acute treatment to reduce relapse and prevent recurrences, but IPT has not shown such effects. Maintenance forms of both CBT and IPT have been developed (e.g., using "booster" sessions once a month) to prevent loss of therapeutic effect, but these have yet to be systematically evaluated. Sequential application of CBT following treatment with antidepressants has also shown benefits in converting partial remitters to full remitters, helping to discontinue antidepressants, and preventing relapse after stopping medications.

Key references

Beck AT, Rush AJ, Shaw BF, et al. Cognitive Therapy of Depression. New York: Guilford Press, 1979.

DeRubeis RJ, Hollon SD, Amsterdam JD, et al. Cognitive therapy vs medications in the treatment of moderate to severe depression. Arch Gen Psychiatry 2005; **62**:409–16.

Dimidjian S, Hollon SD, Dobson KS, et al. Randomized trial of behavioural activation, cognitive therapy, and antidepressant medication in the acute treatment of adults with major depression. J Consult Clin Psychol 2006; **74**:658–70.

Frank E, Grochocinski VJ, Spanier CA, et al. Interpersonal psychotherapy and antidepressant medication: evaluation of a sequential treatment strategy in women with recurrent major depression. J Clin Psychiatry 2000; **61**:51–7.

Hollon SD, DeRubeis RJ, Shelton RC, et al. Prevention of relapse following cognitive therapy vs medications in moderate to severe depression. Arch Gen Psychiatry 2005; **62**:417–22.

Hollon SD, Jarrett RB, Nierenberg AA, et al. Psychotherapy and medication in the treatment of adult and geriatric depression: which monotherapy or combined treatment? J Clin Psychiatry 2005; **66**:455–68.

Keller MB, McCullough JP, Klein DN, et al. A comparison of nefazodone, the cognitive behavioural-analysis system of psychotherapy, and their combination for the treatment of chronic depression. N Engl J Med 2000; **342**:1462–70.

Klerman GL, Weissman MM, Rounsaville BJ, et al. Interpersonal Psychotherapy of Depression. New York: Basic Books, 1984.

Lau MA, Mc Main SF. Integrating mindfulness meditation with cognitive and behavioural therapies: the challenge of combining acceptance- and change-based strategies. Can J Psychiatry 2005; **50**:863–9.

Malouff JM, Thorsteinsson EB, Schutte NS. The efficacy of problem solving therapy in reducing mental and physical health problems: a meta-analysis. Clin Psychol Rev 2007; **27**:46–57.

McCullough JP. *Treatment of Chronic Depression (CBASP)*. New York: Guilford Press, 2000.

Segal ZV, Kennedy SH, Cohen NL. Clinical guidelines for the treatment of depressive disorders. V. Combining psychotherapy and pharmacotherapy. *Can J Psychiatry* 2001; **46**(Suppl 1):59S–62S.

Segal ZV, Whitney DK, Lam RW. Clinical guidelines for the treatment of depressive disorders. III. Psychotherapy. *Can J Psychiatry* 2001; **46**(Suppl 1): 29S–37S.

Weissman MM, Markowitz JC, Klerman GL. *A Comprehensive Guide to Interpersonal Psychotherapy*. New York: Basic Books, 2000.

Wright JH, Wright AS, Albano AM, *et al.* Computer-assisted cognitive therapy for depression: maintaining efficacy while reducing therapist time. *Am J Psychiatry* 2005; 162:1158–64.

Chapter 9

Special populations

> **Key points**
>
> - The keys to optimal management of treatment-resistant depression and depression in special populations include careful assessment, selection of evidence-based treatments tailored to the individual, and ongoing monitoring of response and outcome.
> - Given the still limited evidence base, use and selection of antidepressants depends on an individual risk–benefit assessment in elderly patients, those with other medical illnesses, pregnant and breastfeeding women, and children and adolescents.

9.1 Treatment-resistant depression

9.1.1 Definition and assessment

While most patients with depression respond to initial treatment, up to one-third will not show a clinical response and another 20–30% may not achieve full remission of symptoms. There is unfortunately little high-quality evidence available on how best to manage patients with limited or partial responses, and even less information on optimal sequencing of treatments. Thus, clinical management for these situations is often based only on expert opinion and consensus.

Treatment-resistant depression (TRD) is the term used to describe limited response after several treatments (usually pharmacotherapy). The most commonly used definition for TRD is failure to demonstrate a clinical response to adequate trials of two or more antidepressants, usually from different classes. Clinical response is typically defined as 50% or greater reduction from baseline score using a depression rating scale. An adequate trial usually means that antidepressant treatment has been "optimized" by increasing the dose to the maximum approved dose (or until limited by side effects) for at least 4–6 weeks of treatment. However, this definition of TRD does not take into account partial responses or residual symptoms and, by assuming the first strategy for poor response is switching to another monotherapy, it does not capture failure of other strategies such as augmentation and combination. Hence, findings from studies of TRD may not be generalizable to patients with limited treatment response seen in clinical practice.

Box 9.1 Evaluation for patients with depression who are not responding to treatment

- Reassess adherence to treatment (side effects, taking medication properly, etc.).
- Reassess the diagnosis (especially hypomania, psychotic or seasonal depression, primary dysthymia).
- Reassess for comorbidity (especially anxiety disorder, substance abuse, personality disorder, physical conditions).
- Reassess medication profile (any drug–drug interactions?).
- Determine degree of response/non-response (using a rating scale).
- Consider psychotherapy options.
- Consider pharmacotherapy options.
- Consider electroconvulsive therapy.

The evaluation of patients with TRD involves reassessment of diagnostic and treatment/adherence issues (Box 9.1). Psychoeducation and self-management should be encouraged (see Chapter 5) and an effort to identify psychological targets for intervention may also be beneficial at this stage. Because there is limited information on approaches to the patient who has not responded to psychotherapy, the rest of this section will focus on pharmacotherapy strategies for TRD.

9.1.2 **Pharmacotherapy strategies**

Pharmacotherapy strategies for TRD include switching (to another antidepressant monotherapy), augmenting (adding another medication that by itself is not an antidepressant), and combining (adding a second antidepressant). Often, the terms augmenting and combining are used interchangeably. Augmentation/combination has many potential advantages compared to monotherapy switches, but there are also disadvantages (Table 9.1). Although it may seem that side effects should be higher when two drugs are used, combining can often be done using lower doses of each drug, so the total side effect burden may actually be less than with a high dose of a single drug.

Unfortunately, there is still limited evidence to support efficacy for many of these strategies, and even less information on sequencing of strategies (Table 9.2). However, using a systematic approach (e.g., the Texas Medication Algorithm) with careful documentation and evaluation of response can lead to improved outcomes. Switching from one SSRI to another seems to have a similar efficacy to switching to another class, perhaps because these medications have differences in secondary binding properties. For tips on switching and discontinuing antidepressants, see Chapter 6.

Table 9.1 Advantages and disadvantages of pharmacotherapy strategies for TRD

Strategy	Advantages	Disadvantages
Switch to monotherapy with another antidepressant	• Simple • Better adherence • May be cheaper* • May have fewer side effects* • No drug interactions	• May lose partial benefits of first medication • Possible discontinuation symptoms from stopping first medication • Lag time to response with second medication
Augment or combine with another medication/antidepressant	• Retains therapeutic optimism (by not "giving up" on the first medication) • Allows longer time on first medication • Builds on partial responses • Faster response than with switching • May be able to target specific residual symptoms • May be able to treat side effects of first medication • No problem with discontinuation symptoms	• When combining, never sure if the second antidepressant would have worked by itself • May have more side effects* • May have drug interactions • May be more expensive*

* depends on doses and medications used.

Most clinicians prefer to augment/combine rather than switch when there is partial response to the first medication, in order to not lose any benefits from the first medication. Lithium has the best evidence for augmentation effects, although primarily in augmenting TCAs. Initial studies suggested that low dose lithium augmentation (300–600 mg/day) was beneficial for TRD, but most subsequent studies have shown that lithium dosing to achieve therapeutic serum levels (0.5–1.0 meq/l) are required.

Triiodothyronine has fewer side effects and is easier to use than lithium, and comparative studies show similar efficacy to lithium. Atypical antipsychotics, such as olanzapine, risperidone, and quetiapine, also have shown good evidence as augmentation agents. Another advantage of augmenting/combining is that it may be possible to target specific symptoms or side effects with the second agent. For example, atypical antipsychotics may be particularly beneficial for residual

Table 9.2 Evidence for pharmacotherapy strategies for TRD

Strategy	Medications(s)	Level of evidence*
Switch	• Within same class (SSRIs)	• Level 2
	• To another class	• Level 2
Augment	• Lithium	• Level 1
	• Triiodothyronine	• Level 1
	• Atypical antipsychotics	• Level 1
	• Buspirone	• Level 2
	• Modafinil	• Level 2
	• Psychostimulants	• Level 3
Combine	• SSRI with mirtazapine/mianserin	• Level 1
	• SSRI/SNRI with bupropion	• Level 2
	• SSRI with TCA (caution with CYP 2D6 interactions)	• Level 2
	• SSRI with moclobemide (caution with potential serotonin syndrome)	• Level 3

* Level 1: large, placebo-controlled replicated RCTs, or meta-analysis;
Level 2: at least one RCT;
Level 3: uncontrolled or open-label studies;
Level 4: expert opinion.

symptoms of anxiety or insomnia, triiodothyronine for fatigue, the wake-promoting agent, modafinil, for daytime sleepiness, and bupropion for concentration problems (or to treat SSRI-induced sexual dysfunction).

9.1.3 **STAR*D (Sequenced treatment alternatives to relieve depression)**

STAR*D is an important, large-scale ($N = 3,671$ patients), pragmatic effectiveness study funded by the National Institute of Mental Health in the United States which was designed to provide information on sequencing of treatments for major depressive disorder (MDD) after non-remission with a standard antidepressant (12 weeks of citalopram, 20–60 mg/day). STAR*D incorporates many state-of-the-art features including a focus on remission as the primary outcome, use of real-world patients (e.g., without excluding for comorbidity or substance abuse/dependence) from primary care and specialist settings, large sample size, incorporation of patient preference, and use of measurement-based care. Various levels of treatment were studied, with non-remitters progressing to the next step corresponding to increasing treatment resistance. Although patients could select the sub-study for participation at each level, they were randomized to treatments within the sub-study.

Table 9.3 summarizes the overall results. The remission rates were lower than seen in efficacy RCTs, because the patient population was chronic and challenging to treat. About two-thirds of the patients achieved full remission after four treatment levels. Most of the treatment options were not distinguishable from each other, but unfortunately by Step 3 the sample sizes were too small to detect meaningful differences. There were some differences in tolerability of treatments, for example, citalopram combined with bupropion was better tolerated than when combined with buspirone; triiodothyronine was better tolerated than lithium augmentation. The sub-study with cognitive therapy was smaller than expected, but the remission rates were similar to those of medication options. Overall, this study shows that remission is achievable for the majority of patients, even those with challenging MDD, with increasing intensity of treatments. However, there are still unresolved questions about the comparative efficacy of many of the treatment options studied.

Table 9.3 Summary of STAR*D results			
Level and sample size	**Sub-studies and intervention(s)**	**Remission rate[†, ‡] (%)**	**Cumulative remission[‡] (%)**
Step 1 N = 3,671	• Citalopram	36.8	36.8
Step 2[§] N = 1,439	• SWITCH to: venlafaxine or bupropion or sertraline • COMBINE citalopram with: bupropion or buspirone • SWITCH to or COMBINE with: cognitive therapy	30.6	56.1
Step 3[§] N = 390	• SWITCH to: nortriptyline or mirtazapine • AUGMENT with: lithium or triiodothyronine	13.7	62.1
Step 4 N = 123	• SWITCH to: tranylcypromine or mirtazapine plus venlafaxine	13.0	67.0

† Combined remission rates from all sub-studies within treatment level.
‡ By QIDS-SR criteria.
§ Patients could choose the sub-study for participation, but were randomized to treatments within the sub-study.

9.2 **Elderly and medically ill**

9.2.1 **Diagnostic issues**

There are many similarities in diagnosing and treating depression in the elderly and medically ill populations. Mood disorders in the geriatric age group are frequently precipitated by medical illness and are associated with an increased risk of mortality and longer hospital stays; up to one-half of hospitalized elderly patients have depression. Common treatment considerations include age- and disease-related pharmacokinetic changes, potential drug–drug interactions resulting from polypharmacy, increased sensitivity to side effects, and difficulty differentiating side effects from physical symptoms of the medical condition.

Dementia in elderly patients can present with similar symptoms to MDD (e.g., apathy, psychomotor retardation, etc.). A thorough history and evaluation that examines the onset, course, duration, and treatment response of an individual can help to differentiate between MDD and dementia. The repeated use of cognitive function tests (e.g., mini-mental state exam) can help to distinguish between depression and dementia. For example, early dementia often presents with gradually declining cognitive function whereas individuals with a major depressive episode often show an abrupt cognitive decline coinciding with the onset of depressive symptoms. However, depression and dementia can also co-exist, and the progressing symptoms of dementia subsequently can mask the depressive symptoms (e.g., psychomotor retardation masking decreased concentration).

Numerous studies have also demonstrated that MDD is more common in medically ill individuals compared with the general population (Figure 9.1), but it is both under-diagnosed and under-treated. A common barrier to diagnosis is the mistaken notion that "reactive depression" is not pathological and that treatment is unnecessary or ineffective. Reluctance to stigmatize patients with a psychiatric diagnosis may also play a role. Diagnosis is further complicated by the difficulty in differentiating neurovegetative symptoms of depression (e.g., poor sleep, loss of energy and appetite, fatigue) from physiological symptoms associated with the medical condition. Some screening tools such as the Hospital Anxiety and Depression Scale (HADS, see Appendix) have tried to simplify this by focusing on cognitive symptoms of depression.

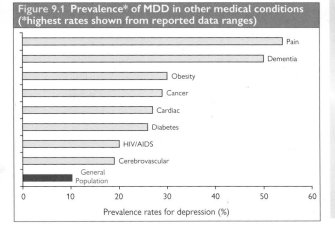

Figure 9.1 Prevalence* of MDD in other medical conditions (*highest rates shown from reported data ranges)

9.2.2 Pharmacotherapy issues

Meta-analyses have shown that pharmacotherapy is safe and generally well-tolerated for MDD in the elderly and in those with various medical illnesses. The maxim, "Start low, go slow, keep going, stay longer" can be applied for the use of antidepressants in these populations (Box 9.2). To minimize side effects, it is generally advisable to begin with a low dosage and gradually titrate up according to clinical response. However, full therapeutic doses of the medications are usually required, although a slower treatment response may be seen. In addition, comorbidity and older age are risk factors for relapse with discontinuation of antidepressants, so maintenance treatment of 2 years or longer is recommended (see Chapter 6).

Selection of antidepressants requires consideration of safety, side effect, and drug-interaction issues (Box 9.2). TCAs and SSRIs are effective in these populations, but TCAs are considered to have a greater side effect burden due to anticholinergic, antihistaminic, and cardiovascular effects. However, these patients may also have difficulty tolerating some of the second-generation antidepressants, for example, gastrointestinal side effects of SSRIs. SSRIs are also associated with hyponatremia in some patients, which may be particularly problematic for the elderly, and with a small increased risk of falls (not due to orthostatic hypotension). Overall, however, SSRIs are still considered first-line antidepressants for elderly and medically ill patients.

> **Box 9.2 Antidepressant selection in the elderly or medically ill**
>
> - Avoid antidepressants that have potential safety issues that interact with the medical illness, e.g., arrhythmogenic and hypotensive effects of TCAs in cardiac patients.
> - Avoid antidepressants with side effects that may worsen symptoms of the medical illness, e.g., venlafaxine in hypertension, mirtazapine or TCAs in diabetes.
> - Avoid antidepressants that may interact with other drugs that patients may be using for the medical illness, e.g., fluvoxamine with warfarin, fluoxetine and paroxetine with codeine; TCAs with quinidine.
> - Be aware of age- and illness-related changes in pharmacokinetics, e.g., liver disease and hepatic dysfunction may reduce metabolism and increase serum levels of antidepressants.
> - "Start low, go slow, keep going, stay longer": start with lower than usual doses, titrate up slowly to usual therapeutic doses, and maintain on medications for a longer duration.

Electroconvulsive therapy (ECT) can be the treatment of choice for some medically ill and elderly patients because it is fast acting and bypasses the problem of medication side effects and interactions. For example, the depressed elder with inability or refusal to eat or drink may have physical deterioration that requires rapid treatment with ECT (see Chapter 7).

9.2.3 **Psychotherapy issues**

Despite the advances being made in psychopharmacology, psychotherapy remains an integral part of managing depression in medically ill patients. Some goals of psychotherapy include improving self-esteem, correcting misconceptions about the illness, and facilitating expression of fears and concerns. It should also enable patients to acknowledge their physical limitations and eventually accept loss and disability. Family therapy is often necessary to expedite communication, prepare the family for change, and alleviate guilt and shame in both parties. Group therapy can decrease social isolation and help patients find meaning in life, despite their illness.

Evidence-based psychotherapies such as CBT and IPT have been demonstrated to be beneficial in many comorbid conditions, including cancer, HIV/AIDS, and cardiovascular disease. As well, CBT and self-management are now widely used in chronic disease management programs as well as for adjunctive treatment of many medical conditions (e.g., insomnia, cancer, diabetes, arthritis, fibromyalgia), even when MDD is not comorbid.

9.2.4 **Depression and cardiovascular disease**

Recent attention has focused on the relationship between MDD and cardiac disease and several recent large clinical trials have been conducted, so it is useful to consider this as an example of medical comorbidity. Up to 25% of patients with angiographic evidence of coronary artery disease will meet criteria for MDD. Indeed, depression is now recognized as an independent risk factor for sudden cardiovascular death, comparable to any of the traditional cardiac risk factors, such as obesity, tobacco use, and hypercholesterolemia. Similarly, 20% of patients surviving a myocardial infarction (MI) will also have a depressive disorder. The mortality risk following MI is 5.7 times higher when MDD is present, making depression a greater risk factor for death post-MI than other cardiac factors such as smoking, history of previous MI, and poor left ventricular function. Several mechanisms have been proposed to explain the relationship of depression to cardiovascular disease and mortality (Table 9.4).

Several large clinical trials have been conducted in patients with cardiac disease and MDD. Two examined patients with MDD who were post-MI. The SAD-HART study showed efficacy of sertraline in improving depression symptoms compared to placebo, while the ENRICH-D study found that cognitive-behavioural therapy (CBT, augmented by sertraline when depression was severe or with non-response after 5 weeks) was modestly effective in reducing depression scores compared to usual care (which may have included antidepressants). The CREATE trial examined citalopram, interpersonal psychotherapy (IPT), and the combination in patients with coronary artery disease. Citalopram was superior to placebo, but IPT alone was not, and the combination was not significantly better than citalopram.

These studies show that SSRIs like citalopram and sertraline are safe and effective for patients with cardiovascular disease, and that CBT (but not IPT) also has benefits. Unfortunately, while all were large sample trials for depression studies, none had a large enough sample to detect changes in mortality or cardiac events. Further study is needed to show whether treatment of MDD in these patients will have direct effects on cardiovascular outcomes.

9.3 **Pregnancy and postpartum**

9.3.1 **Prevalence**

Depressive symptoms are commonly experienced by women during pregnancy and following delivery, but the risk for MDD is also high. For example, "postpartum blues" with mild self-limiting depressive symptoms occurs in up to 50% of women, with up to 30% experiencing

Table 9.4 Potential mechanisms to explain the relationship between depression and cardiovascular mortality and morbidity

Behavioural	Physiological
• Poor concentration and adherence to medication regimens.	• Hyperactivity of the HPA axis, resulting in elevated catecholamine secretion with detrimental effects on the heart, blood vessels and platelets.
• Lack of motivation to adhere to lifestyle changes (e.g., good diet, exercise).	• Augmented platelet responsiveness or activation, increasing the risk of clot formation and atherosclerosis.
• Increased prevalence of habits with negative health consequences (e.g., smoking, binge-eating).	• Altered $5\text{-}HT_2$ receptor density on platelets, thereby increasing platelet aggregation and coronary artery vasoconstriction.
• Reduced activity and social isolation/anxiety making it more difficult to participate in rehabilitation programs.	• Disrupted circadian rhythms and reduced heart rate variability, leading to arrhythmogenesis.

postpartum MDD (see also Chapter 4). Postpartum psychosis, a severe condition requiring emergency treatment, is less common, occurring in 2 out of 1,000 deliveries. Risk factors for postpartum depression include a previous history of postpartum depression, previous history of MDD, depressive symptoms during pregnancy, positive family history, and poor social supports and relationships. Given the high prevalence, screening for depression has been recommended for all women in the postpartum period; the Edinburgh Postnatal Depression Scale (EPDS) has been widely used for both screening and monitoring outcome (see Appendix).

9.3.2 Treatment approaches

There is evidence that non-pharmacological treatments such as IPT and CBT are effective during pregnancy and postpartum, so they should be considered as first-line treatments for MDD. However, there remain significant barriers to access for these evidence-based psychotherapies (see Chapter 8). There is always concern about using medications during pregnancy and postpartum because of potential adverse effects on the fetus and of drug transmission to the infant by breastfeeding. It must be remembered, however, that untreated depression clearly results in poor outcomes for both mother and child, including premature birth, low birth weight, increased neonatal distress, and relationship problems. Discontinuing antidepressants during pregnancy is also not recommended, as the risk of relapse may be as high as 70%.

9.3.3 Antidepressants in pregnancy and breastfeeding

Although the clinical database is not large, the second-generation antidepressants are considered to be relatively safe for use during pregnancy. Fluoxetine is the most widely studied antidepressant in pregnancy. Meta-analyses have shown that the risk for major malformations in women taking most SSRIs (citalopram, escitalopram, fluoxetine, sertraline) is no higher than the base rate of 1–3%. However, first-trimester exposure to paroxetine, particularly at doses higher than 25 mg/day, is associated with a small increased risk of cardiac defects.

Exposure to SSRIs (and other antidepressant classes) is associated with a small increase in the rate of spontaneous abortions, although it is still unclear whether depression itself contributes to this risk. The use of SSRIs in the third trimester is also associated with a transient adaptation syndrome in 10–30% of neonates (compared to 3–10% in non-exposed neonates), consisting of jitteriness, shivering, increased muscle tone, agitation, and mild respiratory distress. The cause of these symptoms is not known, but it may be related to discontinuation effects, as resolution usually occurs within 2 weeks. In regards to longer term effects on infants, two studies have examined neurodevelopmental measures (language, IQ, distractibility, behaviour problems) in children aged 16–86 months after exposure to fluoxetine in utero. Neither found any differences compared to unexposed children of mothers without depression.

Antidepressants are variably excreted in breast milk. Serum levels were undetectable or negligible in infants whose mothers were taking paroxetine, sertraline, and nortriptyline. Maternal use of fluoxetine does lead to detectable serum levels in infants, while the data are inconsistent for citalopram. However, there have been no behavioural effects noted in infants with low serum levels of antidepressants.

In summary, paroxetine has been associated with more neonatal problems than other medications but other SSRIs appear to be safe in pregnancy, although neonates should be monitored for adaptation syndrome. Most antidepressants show low rates of transmission to infants via breast milk, but therapeutic drug monitoring in the infant may be reassuring to mothers as most will have no detectable drug levels. Given the limited database, selection of medication for women in pregnancy and postpartum is still based on an individualized risk–benefit assessment.

9.4 **Children and adolescents**

9.4.1 **Treatment controversies**

Of recent there has been considerable media, public, and professional controversy about the treatment of depression in youth (children and adolescents), centered on the question of antidepressants causing suicidality. This is a complex issue because suicidal thoughts and behaviours are intimately associated with the underlying condition, making it difficult to tease out the relationship between a worsening symptom and medication side effects (Box 9.3, see also Chapter 5).

To further complicate the treatment issue, there are fewer studies on psychosocial treatments for depressed youth compared to adult populations. Unlike childhood anxiety disorders, where there is excellent evidence for efficacy of psychotherapy, there is only limited information about the efficacy of CBT and IPT in youth with depression. While generally positive, many of the studies did not enroll patients with MDD and most were in samples with milder severity. In the one trial with a more severe and comorbid study sample, the Treatment of Adolescents with Depression Study (TADS), CBT was no better than pill placebo while fluoxetine was significantly superior to both. However, there was indication that the best outcomes were achieved with combination fluoxetine and CBT.

9.4.2 **Safety and efficacy of antidepressants**

Previous studies had shown that TCAs were not effective in youth with MDD, but several individual studies with SSRIs found evidence for efficacy of fluoxetine, sertraline, and citalopram. However, when both published and unpublished studies of SSRIs and SNRIs were pooled, the overall effects were non-significant, with only fluoxetine showing significant benefits against placebo. The estimated effect size showed that an excess of 20–25 patients will respond for every 100 patients treated with fluoxetine instead of placebo.

Given the apparent overall lack of benefit of the newer antidepressants, the issue of safety became even more important. Initial meta-analyses conducted by the US Food and Drug Administration (FDA) of published and unpublished RCTs showed small but statistically significant increased risks of suicidality (worsening suicidal thoughts and/or attempts) with newer antidepressants compared to placebo. Of individual drugs, only venlafaxine carried a significantly higher risk, while paroxetine had a trend to significance. Of note is that there were no deaths by suicide within the entire FDA RCT database.

However, a subsequent meta-analysis found different results. Using updated reports from both the FDA and the UK Medicine and Healthcare Products Regulatory Agency which included 3 additional RCTs, the newer antidepressants showed clear superiority versus placebo in MDD and anxiety disorders. The pooled risk difference for achieving clinical response in MDD was 11%, with a Number Needed to Treat (NNT) of 10, indicating that 10 patients need to be treated with antidepressants to gain one more patient in clinical response compared to using placebo.

Additionally, the risk of suicidality of antidepressants based on all trials for all conditions (including anxiety disorders) was still significantly higher than for placebo, but the risk was smaller than previous; however, in studies of MDD the suicidality risk was no longer statistically significant. The Number Needed to Harm (NNH) was estimated at 112, which means that 112 patients need to be treated with an antidepressant before finding one additional patient with suicidality compared to using placebo.

The individual RCTs (other than TADS) have been critiqued because of high placebo responses, low severity of patients, and limited generalizability of results. Other types of studies have not supported increased suicidality, with antidepressants in youth. For example, database studies of naturalistic treatment have not found greatly increased risks for suicidality; toxicology studies have shown that youths that die by suicide do not show presence of SSRIs in their blood, and pharmacoepidemiology studies show that increasing prescription rates for SSRIs are associated with declining suicide rates, which would not be expected if suicide was associated with antidepressants.

Box 9.3 Potential causes for worsening suicidality when starting an antidepressant

- Worsening of depression in the natural course of illness, as patients generally come to attention when the severity of their depression is highest.
- Initial improvement in physical symptoms of depression (e.g., energy) before cognitive symptoms (e.g., hopelessness), so that suicidal thoughts can be actualized.
- Unforeseen psychosocial stressor (e.g., breakup of relationship, family conflict).
- Demoralization from lack of treatment response.
- Non-specific side effects of antidepressant (e.g., nausea, insomnia) causing increased worry and anxiety.
- Specific side effects of antidepressant (e.g., agitation, activation syndrome).
- Antidepressant-induced hypomania or mixed state in a patient with an unrecognized bipolar disorder.

> **Box 9.4 Recommendations for children and adolescents with MDD**
>
> - For MDD of mild to moderate severity, evidence-based psycho-therapy (CBT or IPT) alone should be used, whenever possible.
> - For MDD of marked or worse severity, antidepressants are indicated. Fluoxetine is the only first-line antidepressant recommended because of its proven efficacy and safety profile. Combining with psychotherapy may also improve efficacy and reduce risk of medication-associated suicidality.
> - Other SSRIs such as citalopram and sertraline, despite slightly increased risk of worsening suicidality, can be used as second-line treatments, especially when depression is severe, chronic, associated with comorbidity, and when psychosocial treatments have not helped.
> - Other novel agents (agomelatine, bupropion, mirtazapine) are considered third-line medications because of limited evidence for efficacy or side effect burden.
> - TCAs, venlafaxine, paroxetine, and duloxetine are not recommended based on lack of evidence for efficacy and increased risk for suicidality.
> - Close monitoring (e.g., at least weekly contact for the first month of treatment) for treatment response and suicidality is important, particularly in the early phases of treatment when the suicide risk is highest.
> - Discussion with patient and family about potential side effects should be done prior to initiation of treatment (e.g., suicidality, agitation, anxiety, irritability, hypomania and activation syndrome)

In summary, newer antidepressants do show benefit in MDD and can be used in youth, but cautiously and with careful evaluation of risk–benefit for individual patients (Box 9.4). There is a suggestion of a small risk of suicidality based on placebo-controlled RCTs, but little additional evidence to corroborate this finding. Regardless, it is possible that antidepressants worsen suicidality in a small subset of vulnerable patients, so it is prudent to carefully monitor patients, particularly early in treatment when they are at highest risk for suicide.

Key references

Beliles K, Stoudemire A. Psychopharmacologic treatment of depression in the medically ill. *Psychosomatics* 1998; **39**:S2–S19.

Bridge JA, Iyengar S, Salary CB, *et al.* Clinical response and risk for reported suicidal ideation and suicide attempts in paediatric antidepressants treatment: a meta-analysis of randomized controlled trials. *JAMA* 2007; **297**:1683–96.

Einarson TR, Einarson A. Newer antidepressants in pregnancy and rates of major malformations: a metaanalysis of prospective comparative studies. *Pharmacoepidemiol Drug Saf* 2005; **14**: 823–27.

Evans DL, Charney DS, Lewis L, *et al.* Mood disorders in the medically ill: scientific review and recommendations. *Biol Psychiatry* 2005; **58**:175–89.

Evans DL, Staab JP, Petitto JM, *et al.* Depression in the medical setting: biopsychological interactions and treatment considerations. *J Clin Psychiatry* 1999; **60**(Suppl 4):40–55.

Fava M. Diagnosis and definition of treatment resistant depression. *Biol Psychiatry* 2003; 53:649–59.

Gill D, Hatcher S. Antidepressants for depression in people with physical illness. *Cochrane Database Syst Rev* 2000; **4**:CD001312

Hammad TA, Laughren T, Racoosin J. Suicidality in paediatric patients treated with antidepressant drugs. *Arch Gen Psychiatry* 2006; **63**:332–9.

Kennedy SH, Lam RW, Cohen NL, *et al.* Clinical guidelines for the treatment of depressive disorders. IV. Medications and other biological treatments. *Can J Psychiatry* 2001; **46**(Suppl. 1):38S–58S.

Lam RW, Kennedy SH. Prescribing antidepressants for depression in 2005: recent concerns and recommendations. *Can J Psychiatry* 2005; **49**(Insert):1–6.

March J, Silva S, Petrycki S, *et al.* Fluoxetine, cognitive-behavioural therapy, and their combination for adolescents with depression: treatment for Adolescents with Depression Study (TADS) randomized controlled trial. *JAMA* 2004; **292**:807–20.

Nulman I, Rovet J. Stewart DE, *et al.* Child development following exposure to tricyclic antidepressants or fluoxetine throughout foetal life: a prospective controlled study. *Am J Psychiatry* 2002; 159:1889–95.

Rush AJ, Trivedi MH, Wisniewski SR, *et al.* Acute and longer-term outcomes in depressed outpatients requiring one or several treatment steps: a STAR*D report. *Am J Psychiatry* 2006; 163:1905–17.

Souery D, Papakostas GJ, Trivedi MH. Treatment-resistant depression. *J Clin Psychiatry* 2006; **67**(Suppl 6):16–22.

Stewart DE. Antidepressant drugs during pregnancy and lactation. *Int Clin Psychopharmacol* 2000; **15**(Suppl 3):S19–S24.

Thorpe L, Whitney DK, Kutcher SP, *et al.* Clinical guidelines for the treatment of depressive disorders. VI. Special populations. *Can J Psychiatry* 2001; **46**(Suppl 1):63S–78S.

Vasa RA, Carlino AR, Pine DS. Pharmacotherapy of depressed children and adolescents: current issues and potential directions. *Biol Psychiatry* 2006; **59**:1021–28.

Way CM. Safety of newer antidepressants in pregnancy. *Pharmacotherapy* 2007; 27:546–52.

Wisner KL, Parry BL, Piontek CM. Clinical practice. Postpartum depression. *N Engl J Med* 2002; **347**:194–9.

Appendix

Appendix

Sample rating scales

Rating scale	Key features/limitations	Done by	Length and time
Hamilton Depression Rating Scale (HAM-D, HDRS)	Most widely used outcome measure in clinical trials, not all DSM-IV symptoms covered.	Clinician	17–24 items 20–30 min
Montgomery-Asberg Depression Rating Scale (MADRS)	Widely used in clinical trials, specialized training not required, sensitive to change, not all DSM-IV symptoms covered.	Clinician	10 items, 15 min
Quick Inventory of Depressive Symptomatology, Self-Rated (QIDS-SR)	Used in the STAR*D effectiveness trial, all DSM-IV symptoms covered.	Patient	17 items, 10 min
Patient Health Questionnaire (PHQ-9)	Brief, validated in primary care settings, follows the DSM-IV symptom criteria, useful for screening, diagnosis and monitoring outcomes.	Patient	9 items, 5 min
Hospital Anxiety and Depression Scale (HADS)	Screening tool for medically ill patients, validated in hospital and primary care settings, not all DSM-IV-symptoms covered.	Patient	14 items, 5 min
Edinburgh Postnatal Depression Scale (EPDS)	Screens for postpartum depression, validated in primary care settings not all DSH-IV symptoms covered.	Patient	10 items, 20 min

Key references

Cox J, Holden J, Sagovsky R. Detection of postnatal depression. Development of the 10-item Edinburgh Postnatal Depression Scale. *Br J Psychiatry* 1987; **150**: 782–6.

Hamilton M. Development of a rating scale for primary depressive illness. *Br J Soc Clin Psych* 1967; **6**: 278–96.

Kroenke K, Spitzer RL, Williams JB. The PHQ–9: validity of a brief depression severity measure. *J Gen Intern Med* 2001; **16**: 606–13.

Lam RW, Michalak EE, Swinson RP: Assessment Scales in Depression, Mania and Anxiety. London: Taylor and Francis, 2005.

Montgomery SA, Asberg M. A new depression scale designed to be sensitive to change. *Br J Psychiatry* 1979; **134**: 382–9.

Trivedi MH, Rush AJ, Ibrahim HM, et al. The Inventory of Depressive Symptomatology, Clinician Rating (IDS-C) and Self-Report (IDS-SR), and the Quick Inventory of Depressive Symptomatology, Clinician Rating (QIDS-C) and Self-Report (QIDS-SR) in public sector patients with mood disorders: a psychometric evaluation. *Psychol Med* 2004; **34**: 73–82.

Wilkinson MJ, Barczak P. Psychiatric screening in general practice: comparison of the general health questionnaire and the hospital anxiety depression scale. *J R Coll Gen Pract* 1988; **38**: 311–13.

Hamilton Depression Rating Scale, 17-item version (Ham-D, HDRS)

1. Depressed mood

0 = Absent.
1 = These feeling states indicated only on questioning.
2 = These feeling states spontaneously reported verbally.
3 = Communicates feeling states non-verbally—i.e., through facial expression, posture, voice, and tendency to weep.
4 = Patient reports virtually only these feeling states in his spontaneous verbal and non-verbal communication.

2. Work and activities

0 = No difficulty.
1 = Thoughts and feelings of incapacity, fatigue or weakness related to activities; work or hobbies.
2 = Loss of interest in activities; hobbies or work—either directly reported by patient, or indirect in listlessness, indecision and vacillation (feels he has to push self to work or activities).
3 = Decrease in actual time spent in activities or decrease in productivity. In hospital rate 3 if patient does not spend at least 3 h a day in activities (hospital job or hobbies) exclusive of ward chores.
4 = Stopped working because of present illness. In hospital, rate 4 if patient engages in no activities except ward chores, or if patient fails to perform ward chores unassisted.

3. Genital symptoms

0 = Absent.
1 = Mild.
2 = Severe.

4. Somatic symptoms—GI

0 = None.
1 = Loss of appetite but eating without staff encouragement. Heavy feelings in abdomen.
2 = Difficulty eating without staff urging. Requests or requires laxatives or medication for bowels or medication for G.I. symptoms.

5. Loss of weight

0 = No weight loss.
1 = Probable weight loss associated with present illness.
2 = Definite (according to patient) weight loss.

6. Insomnia—early

0 = No difficulty falling asleep.
1 = Complains or occasional difficulty falling asleep—i.e., more than 1/2 h.
2 = Complains of nightly difficulty falling asleep.

7. Insomnia—middle

0 = No difficulty.
1 = Patient complains of being restless and disturbed during the night.
2 = Waking during the night—any getting out of bed rates 2 (except for purposes of voiding).

8. Insomnia—late

0 = No difficulty.
1 = Waking in early hours of the morning but goes back to sleep.
2 = Unable to fall asleep again if he gets out of bed.

9. Somatic symptoms—general

0 = None.
1 = Heaviness in limbs, back or head. Backaches, headache, muscle aches. Loss of energy and fatigability.
2 = Any clear-cut symptom rates 2.

10. Feelings of guilt

0 = Absent.
1 = Self reproach, feels he has let people down.
2 = Ideas of guilt or rumination over past errors or sinful deeds.
3 = Present illness is a punishment. Delusions of guilt.
4 = Hears accusatory or denunciatory voices and/or experiences threatening visual hallucinations.

11. Suicide

0 = Absent.
1 = Feels life is not worth living.
2 = Wishes he were dead or any thoughts of possible death to self.
3 = Suicide ideas or gestures.
4 = Attempts at suicide (any serious attempt rates 4).

12. Anxiety—psychic

0 = No difficulty.
1 = Subjective tension and irritability.
2 = Worrying about minor matters.
3 = Apprehensive attitude apparent in face or speech.
4 = Fears expressed without questioning.

13. Anxiety—somatic

0 = Absent.
1 = Mild.
2 = Moderate.
3 = Severe.
4 = Incapacitating.

14. Hypochondriasis

0 = Not present
1 = Self-absorption (bodily).
2 = Preoccupation with health.
3 = Frequent complaints, requests for help, etc.
4 = Hypochondriacal delusions.

15. Insight

0 = Acknowledges being depressed and ill.
1 = Acknowledges illness but attributes cause to bad food, climate, over work, virus, need for rest, etc.
2 = Denies being ill at all.

16. Motor retardation

0 = Normal speech and thought.
1 = Slight retardation at interview.
2 = Obvious retardation at interview.
3 = Interview difficult.
4 = Complete stupor.

17. Agitation

0 = None.
1 = Fidgetiness.
2 = Playing with hands, hair, etc.
3 = Moving about can't sit still.
4 = Hand wringing, nail biting, hair pulling, biting of lips.

17-item HAMD Total: _____

Scoring Criteria	
0–7	Normal (remission)
8–17	Mildly depressed
18–24	Moderately depressed
25 or higher	Severely depressed

Montgomery–Asberg Depression Rating Scale (MADRS)

The rating should be based on a clinical interview moving from broadly phrased questions about symptoms to more detailed ones that allow a precise rating of severity. The rater must decide whether the rating lies on the defined scale steps (0, 2, 4, 6) or between them (1, 3, 5).

Circle the score that best characterizes the patient at this time.

Item	Explanation
1. Apparent sadness	0 No sadness 2 Looks dispirited but does brighten up without difficulty 4 Appears sad and unhappy most of the time 6 Looks miserable all the time. Extremely despondent.
2. Reported sadness	0 Occasional sadness in keeping with the circumstances. 2 Sad or low but brightens up without difficulty. 4 Pervasive feelings of sadness or gloominess. The mood is still influenced by external circumstances. 6 Continuous unvarying sadness, misery or despondency.
3. Inner tension	0 Placid. Only fleeting inner tension. 2 Occasional feelings of edginess and ill-defined discomfort. 4 Continuous feelings of inner tension or intermittent panic that the patient can master only with some difficulty. 6 Unrelenting dread or anguish. Overwhelming panic
4. Reduced sleep	0 Sleeps as usual 2 Slight difficulty dropping off to sleep or slightly reduced, light or fitful sleep. 4 Sleep reduced or broken by at least 2 h. 6 Less than 2 or 3 h sleep.
5. Reduced appetite	0 Normal or increased appetite. 2 Slightly reduced appetite 4 No appetite. Food is tasteless. 6 Needs persuasion to eat.
6. Concentration difficulties	0 No difficulties in concentrating. 2 Occasional difficulties in collecting one's thoughts. 4 Difficulties in concentrating and sustaining thought that reduces ability to read or hold a conversation. 6 Unable to read or converse without great difficulty.

7. Lassitude	0 Hardly any difficulty in getting started. No sluggishness.
	2 Difficulties in starting activities
	4 Difficulties in starting simple routine activities that are carried out with effort.
	6 Complete lassitude. Unable to do anything without help.
8. Inability to feel	0 Normal interest in the surroundings and other people
	2 Reduced ability to enjoy usual interests.
	4 Loss of interest in the surroundings. Loss of feelings for friends and acquaintances.
	6 The experience of being emotionally paralyzed, inability to feel anger, grief, or pleasure and a complete or even painful failure to feel for close relatives and friends.
9. Pessimistic thoughts	0 No pessimistic thoughts.
	2 Fluctuating ideas of failure, self-reproach, or self-depreciation.
	4 Persistent self-accusations, or definite but still rational ideas of guilt, or sin. Increasingly pessimistic about the future.
	6 Delusions of ruin, remorse, or unredeemable sin. Self-accusations which are absurd and unshakable.
10. Suicidal thoughts	0 Enjoys life or takes it as it comes
	2 Weary of life. Only fleeting suicidal thoughts.
	4 Probably better off dead. Suicidal thoughts are common, and suicide is considered as a possible solution, but without specific plans or intention.
	6 Explicit plans for suicide when there is an opportunity. Active preparations for suicide.

TOTAL SCORE _____

Scoring Criteria	
0–12	Normal (remission)
13–19	Mildly depressed
20–29	Moderately depressed
30 or higher	Severely depressed

Quick inventory of depressive symptomatology (self-report) (QIDS-SR)

Please circle the one response to each item that best describes you for the past seven days.

1. Falling Asleep:
0 I never take longer than 30 minutes to fall asleep.
1 I take at least 30 minutes to fall asleep, less than half the time.
2 I take at least 30 minutes to fall asleep, more than half the time.
3 I take more than 60 minutes to fall asleep, more than half the time.

2. Sleep During the Night:
0 I do not wake up at night.
1 I have a restless, light sleep with a few brief awakenings each night.
2 I wake up at least once a night, but I go back to sleep easily.
3 I awaken more than once a night and stay awake for 20 minutes or more, more than half the time.

3. Waking Up Too Early:
0 Most of the time, I awaken no more than 30 minutes before I need to get up.
1 More than half the time, I awaken more than 30 minutes before I need to get up.
2 I almost always awaken at least one hour or so before I need to, but I go back to sleep eventually.
3 I awaken at least one hour before I need to, and can't go back to sleep.

4. Sleeping Too Much:
0 I sleep no longer than 7–8 hours/night, without napping during the day.
1 I sleep no longer than 10 hours in a 24-hour period including naps.
2 I sleep no longer than 12 hours in a 24-hour period including naps.
3 I sleep longer than 12 hours in a 24-hour period including naps.

5. Feeling Sad:
0 I do not feel sad
1 I feel sad less than half the time.
2 I feel sad more than half the time.
3 I feel sad nearly all of the time.

6. Decreased Appetite:
0 There is no change in my usual appetite.
1 I eat somewhat less often or lesser amounts of food than usual.
2 I eat much less than usual and only with personal effort.
3 I rarely eat within a 24-hour period, and only with extreme personal effort or when others persuade me to eat.

7. Increased Appetite:

0 There is no change from my usual appetite.
1 I feel a need to eat more frequently than usual.
2 I regularly eat more often and/or greater amounts of food than usual.
3 I feel driven to overeat both at mealtime and between meals.

8. Decreased Weight (Within the Last Two Weeks):

0 I have not had a change in my weight.
1 I feel as if I've had a slight weight loss.
2 I have lost 2 pounds or more.
3 I have lost 5 pounds or more.

9. Increased Weight (Within the Last Two Weeks):

0 I have not had a change in my weight.
1 I feel as if I've had a slight weight gain.
2 I have gained 2 pounds or more.
3 I have gained 5 pounds or more.

10. Concentration/Decision Making:

0 There is no change in my usual capacity to concentrate or make decisions.
1 I occasionally feel indecisive or find that my attention wanders.
2 Most of the time, I struggle to focus my attention or to make decisions.
3 I cannot concentrate well enough to read or cannot make even minor decisions.

11. View of Myself:

0 I see myself as equally worthwhile and deserving as other people.
1 I am more self-blaming than usual.
2 I largely believe that I cause problems for others.
3 I think almost constantly about major and minor defects in myself.

12. Thoughts of Death or Suicide:

0 I do not think of suicide or death.
1 I feel that life is empty or wonder if it's worth living.
2 I think of suicide or death several times a week for several minutes.
3 I think of suicide or death several times a day in some detail, or have made specific plans for suicide or have actually tried to take my life.

13. General Interest:

0 There is no change from usual in how interested I am in other people or activities.
1 I notice that I am less interested in people or activities.
2 I find I have interest in only one or two of my formerly pursued activities.
3 I have virtually no interest in formerly pursued activities.

14. Energy Level:

0 There is no change in my usual level of energy.
1 I get tired more easily than usual.
2 I have to make a big effort to start or finish my usual daily activities (for example, shopping, homework, cooking or going to work).
3 I really cannot carry out most of my usual daily activities because I just don't have the energy.

15. Feeling slowed down:

0 I think, speak, and move at my usual rate of speed.
1 I find that my thinking is slowed down or my voice sounds dull or flat.
2 It takes me several seconds to respond to most questions and I'm sure my thinking is slowed.
3 I am often unable to respond to questions without extreme effort.

16. Feeling restless:

0 I do not feel restless.
1 I'm often fidgety, wringing my hands, or need to shift how I am sitting.
2 I have impulses to move about and am quite restless.
3 At times, I am unable to stay seated and need to pace around.

To Score:

1. Enter the highest score on any 1 of the 4 sleep items (1–4) ____
2. Item 5 ____
3. Enter the highest score on any 1 appetite/weight item (6–9) ____
4. Item 10 ____
5. Item 11 ____
6. Item 12 ____
7. Item 13 ____
8. Item 14 ____
9. Enter the highest score on either of the 2 psychomotor items (15 and 16) ____

TOTAL SCORE (Range 0–27) ____

Scoring Criteria	
0–5	Normal
6–10	Mild
11–15	Moderate
16–20	Severe
≥21	Very Severe

©2000, A. John Rush, M.D.

Patient Health Questionnaire (PHQ-9)

1. Over the last 2 weeks, how often have you been bothered by any of the following problems?

	Not at all (0)	Several days (1)	More than half the days (2)	Nearly every day (3)
a. Little interest or pleasure in doing things.	☐	☐	☐	☐
b. Feeling down, depressed, or hopeless.	☐	☐	☐	☐
c. Trouble falling/staying asleep, sleeping too much.	☐	☐	☐	☐
d. Feeling tired or having little energy.	☐	☐	☐	☐
e. Poor appetite or overeating.	☐	☐	☐	☐
f. Feeling bad about yourself, or that you are a failure, or have let yourself or your family down.	☐	☐	☐	☐
g. Trouble concentrating on things, such as reading the newspaper or watching TV.	☐	☐	☐	☐
h. Moving or speaking so slowly that other people could have noticed. Or the opposite; being so fidgety or restless that you have been moving around more than usual.	☐	☐	☐	☐
i. Thoughts that you would be better off dead or of hurting yourself in some way.	☐	☐	☐	☐

2. If you checked off any problem on this questionnaire so far, how difficult have these problems made it for you to do your work, take care of things at home, or get along with other people?

☐ Not difficult at all   ☐ Somewhat difficult   ☐ Very difficult   ☐ Extremely difficult

TOTAL SCORE _____

Scoring Criteria	
0–4	Normal (remission)
5–14	Mildly depressed
15–19	Moderately depressed
20 or higher	Severely depressed

Hospital Anxiety and Depression Scale (H.

Doctors are aware that emotions play an important part in most illnesses. If your doctor knows about these feelings he will be able to help you more. This questionnaire is designed to help your doctor to know how you feel. Read each item and place a firm tick in the box opposite the reply that comes closest to how you have been feeling in the past week. Don't take too long over your replies: your immediate reaction to each item will probably be more accurate than a long thought-out response.

Tick only one box in each section

1. I feel tense or wound up:
☐ 3 Most of the time
☐ 2 A lot of the time
☐ 1 Time to time
☐ 0 Not at all

2. I still enjoy the things I used to enjoy:
☐ 0 Definitely as much
☐ 1 Not quite so much
☐ 2 Only a little
☐ 3 Hardly at all

3. I get a sort of frightened feeling as if something awful is about to happen:
☐ 3 Very definitely and quite badly
☐ 2 Yes, but not too badly
☐ 1 A little, but it doesn't worry me
☐ 0 Not at all

4. I can laugh and see the funny side of things:
☐ 0 As much as I always could
☐ 1 Not quite as much now
☐ 2 Definitely not so much now
☐ 3 Not at all

5. Worrying thoughts go through my mind:
☐ 3 A great deal of the time
☐ 2 A lot of the time
☐ 1 From time to time but not too often
☐ 0 Only occasionally

6. I feel cheerful:
☐ 3 Not at all
☐ 2 Not often
☐ 1 Sometimes
☐ 0 Most of the time

7. I can sit at ease and feel relaxed:

☐ 0 Definitely
☐ 1 Usually
☐ 2 Not often
☐ 3 Not at all

8. I feel as if I am slowed down:

☐ 3 Nearly all the time
☐ 2 Very often
☐ 1 Sometimes
☐ 0 Not at all

9. I get a sort of frightened feeling like butterflies in the stomach:

☐ 0 Not at all
☐ 1 Occasionally
☐ 2 Quite often
☐ 3 Very often

10. I have lost interest in my appearance:

☐ 3 Definitely
☐ 2 I don't take so much care as I should
☐ 1 I may not take quite as much care
☐ 0 I take just as much care as ever

11. I feel restless as if I have to be on the move:

☐ 3 Very much indeed
☐ 2 Quite a lot
☐ 1 Not very much
☐ 0 Not at all

12. I look forward with enjoyment to things:

☐ 0 As much as ever I did
☐ 1 Rather less than I used to
☐ 2 Definitely less than I used to
☐ 3 Hardly at all

13. I get sudden feelings of panic:

☐ 3 Very often indeed
☐ 2 Quite often
☐ 1 Not very often
☐ 0 Not at all

14. I can enjoy a good book or radio or TV program:

☐ 0 Often
☐ 1 Sometimes
☐ 2 Not often
☐ 3 Very seldom

Scoring: Even questions are for depression. Odd questions are for anxiety. Score each separately. A score of 8 or more is significant, a score of 11 or more highly significant.

Edinburgh Postnatal Depression Scale (EPDS)

As you have recently had a baby, we would like to know how you are feeling now. Please <u>underline</u> the answer which best describes how you have felt in the past 7 days, not just how you feel today. Here is an ex-ample, already completed:

I have felt happy:
Yes, most the time
<u>Yes, some of the time</u>
No, not very often
No, not at all

This would mean: 'I have felt happy some of the time during the past week'. Please complete the other questions in the same way.

In the past 7 days:

1. I have been able to laugh and see the funny side of things:
As much as I always could
Not quite so much now
Definitely not so much now
Not at all

2. I have looked forward with enjoyment to things:
As much as I ever did
Rather less than I used to
Definitely less than I used to
Hardly at all

3. I have blamed myself unnecessarily when things went wrong:
Yes, most of the time
Yes, some of the time
Not very often
No, never

4. I have been anxious or worried for no good reason:
No, not at all
Hardly ever
Yes, sometimes
Yes, very often

5. I have felt scared or panicky for no very good reason:
Yes, quite a lot
Yes, sometimes
No, not much
No, not at all

6. **Things have been getting on top of me:**
   Yes, most of the time I haven't been able to cope at all
   Yes, sometimes I haven't been coping as well as usual
   No, most of the time I have coped quite well
   No, I have been coping as well as ever

7. **I have been so unhappy that I have had difficulty sleeping:**
   Yes, most of the time
   Yes, sometimes
   Not very often
   No, not at all

8. **I have felt sad or miserable:**
   Yes, most of the time
   Yes, quite often
   Not very often
   No, not at all

9. **I have been so unhappy that I have been crying:**
   Yes, most of the time
   Yes, quite often
   Only occasionally
   No, never

10. **The thought of harming myself has occurred to me:**
    Yes, quite often
    Sometimfs
    Hardly ever
    Never

Translations of the scale, and guidance as to its use, may be found in Cox, J.L. & Holden, J. (2003). *Perinatal Mental Health: A Guide to the Edinburgh Postnatal Depression Scale.* London: Gaskell.

Index